# Clinical Inertia

Gérard Reach

# Clinical Inertia

## A Critique of Medical Reason

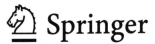

Gérard Reach
Avicenne Hospital and Paris 13 University, Sorbonne Paris Cité
Bobigny
France

Translation from the French language edition 'L'inertie clinique' by Reach, Gérard, © Springer-Verlag France, Paris, 2013; ISBN 978-2-8178-0312-8.
Translation by Claudia Ratti

ISBN 978-3-319-09881-4        ISBN 978-3-319-09882-1   (eBook)
DOI 10.1007/978-3-319-09882-1
Springer Cham Heidelberg New York Dordrecht London

Library of Congress Control Number: 2014951512

© Springer International Publishing Switzerland 2015
This work is subject to copyright. All rights are reserved by the Publisher, whether the whole or part of the material is concerned, specifically the rights of translation, reprinting, reuse of illustrations, recitation, broadcasting, reproduction on microfilms or in any other physical way, and transmission or information storage and retrieval, electronic adaptation, computer software, or by similar or dissimilar methodology now known or hereafter developed. Exempted from this legal reservation are brief excerpts in connection with reviews or scholarly analysis or material supplied specifically for the purpose of being entered and executed on a computer system, for exclusive use by the purchaser of the work. Duplication of this publication or parts thereof is permitted only under the provisions of the Copyright Law of the Publisher's location, in its current version, and permission for use must always be obtained from Springer. Permissions for use may be obtained through RightsLink at the Copyright Clearance Center. Violations are liable to prosecution under the respective Copyright Law.
The use of general descriptive names, registered names, trademarks, service marks, etc. in this publication does not imply, even in the absence of a specific statement, that such names are exempt from the relevant protective laws and regulations and therefore free for general use.
While the advice and information in this book are believed to be true and accurate at the date of publication, neither the authors nor the editors nor the publisher can accept any legal responsibility for any errors or omissions that may be made. The publisher makes no warranty, express or implied, with respect to the material contained herein.

Printed on acid-free paper

Springer is part of Springer Science+Business Media (www.springer.com)

*To Isabelle*

*First law of motion, or principle of inertia:*
*Every body persists in its state of being at rest*
*or of moving uniformly straight forward,*
*except insofar as it is compelled to*
*change its state by force impressed.*
Sir Isaac Newton, Mathematical Principles
of Natural Philosophy (1687)

*Insanity: doing the same thing over*
*and over again*
*and expecting different results.*
Einstein

# Foreword

In this book, and in his other writings on the psychology of the doctor-patient relationship, Dr. Gérard Reach breaks new ground. He does so because he comes to the issues as practicing doctor and as a medical researcher, not as a moral philosopher or cognitive psychologist. He is able, therefore, to identify the questions and problems *that really matter*. I find his bottom-up approach highly attractive. At the same time, Dr. Reach is thoroughly familiar with the relevant philosophical and psychological literature, from the classical writings by Daniel Kahneman, Amos Tversky, George Ainslie and Donald Davidson to the recent work by Roy Baumeister, Walter Mischel, and Pascal Engel.

I shall not attempt to summarize the work, only offer some reflections on it. In doing so, I shall draw not only on the present book, but also on the ideas that Dr. Reach presents in a companion volume, *The Mental Mechanisms of Patient Adherence to Long Term Therapies*. Although his ideas on clinical inertia are briefly presented at the end of the latter book, they are less fully developed than in the present one, which is devoted exclusively to that topic. This book also contains a remarkably sophisticated discussion of evidence-based medicine and its pitfalls.

The basic schema of the analyses in the two books can be presented as follows:

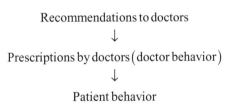

Thus Dr. Reach asks (i) why doctors sometimes do not adhere to the recommendations of medical authorities such as, in France, the Haute Autorité de Santé and, in the United States, the National Guideline Clearinghouse, and (ii) why patients sometimes do not comply with the prescriptions and other recommendations of their doctors. I shall discuss both issues, beginning with the latter.

## Nonadherence by Patients

It might seem that nonadherence by patients to a medical or behavioral regime prescribed to them by their doctors can only be characterized as irrational. They *want* to get better; they *know* what to do to get better; and yet they *don't do it*. In some cases, this characterization seems correct. Patients may fail to take their medication because it reminds them of their mortality, just as people sometimes put off writing a will until it's too late because they don't want to entertain the thought of their death. Anyone can forget to take their medication, but sometimes the forgetfulness is *motivated*. They may fail to do their midday injection because they would feel ashamed to do so in front of their peers. People who are told by their doctor to cut down their wine consumption to two glasses a day, may start using larger glasses; if told not to drink before dinner, they may move up their dinner-time.

In other cases, the epithet "irrational" is less obviously appropriate. As Dr. Reach emphasizes, people may stop taking their medication if it has negative secondary effects that appear before the curative effects *and* the patient is myopic, that is, has a high rate of time preference. In itself, the second factor is not necessarily irrational, at least if one adopts, as I do, a purely subjective conception of rationality (Elster 2007, Ch.11.) A myopic person may act *unwisely*, as judged by an external observer, but that is a different matter. If, however, the patient discounts the future *hyperbolically* (Ainslie 1992), he or she may have a firm intention to abide by the regime only to find her preferences reversed when the time for action arrives. Such behavior is indeed irrational. Yet hyperbolic time discounting is not the only, and probably not the most important, source of preference reversal. As Dr. Reach notes, the initial enthusiasm to fight an illness typically wanes with time. As these energetic but short-lived emotions wane, so does treatment adherence. In this case, the irrationality consists in the failure to understand that the emotion is unlikely to last – the "hot-to-cold empathy gap" (Loewenstein 2005).

The last remark suggests the following question: if patients become aware that they have "an adherence problem", what can they do about it? Let me first use a fanciful example. Dr. Reach refers to the substance Antabus (disulfiram) that some ex-alcoholics take to prevent themselves from backsliding: when taken at the same time as alcohol, it induces vomiting. Suppose now that for a given medication, to be taken once a day, one could invent a substance, to be ingested once a month, so that failure to take the daily medication would induce acute nausea. I assume that this can't be done, but are there any more realistic technologies of self-control available? One possibility would be an automated phone-call, "It is time to take your daily medication". If the doctor has ordained regular physical exercise, the patient can motivate himself by going to a fitness center where he pays a large down payment that is reimbursed in part after each visit.

In his writings Dr. Reach often discusses the idea of patient autonomy, or (roughly speaking) informed consent, and notes that patients sometimes do not want to exercise their autonomy, preferring to leave the decisions in the hand of the doctor. In a variation on a phrase by T. S. Eliot, one might say that humankind cannot bear very much freedom. Some people, though, are obsessed with their freedom and

Foreword xi

autonomy of choice, and hate doing what they are told to do. As Dr. Reach notes, this is the phenomenon of *reactance* that has been observed in many other contexts as well. In his analysis of the psychoanalytic phenomenon of resistance, Lacan (1977, p. 13) refers to "that resistance of *amour-propre*, to use the term in all the depth given to it by La Rochefoucauld, and which is often expresses thus: I can't bear the thought of being freed by anyone other than myself".

Let me mention some sources of rational non-compliance. First, there may be *rational distrust* of the doctor – either of the doctor's *competence* or of his *honesty*. In the case of psychiatric treatment, for instance, the low degree of intersubjective agreement among doctors that belong to different schools of thought would seem to justify skepticism and sometimes nonadherence. Prescription of medication for attention deficit disorder may be an example. In the case of surgeons, their notorious eagerness to operate, sometimes motivated by a financial interest, can justify resistance to their advice. Four years ago, a doctor told me that I needed to have knee surgery immediately, since there was no cartilage left, only "bone on bone". I discarded the advice, and instead lost weight, resumed biking, and am doing just fine. In such cases, one might want to seek a second opinion – but not tell the second doctor what the first doctor concluded!

The mirror image of rational distrust is that of *irrational trust*. When deciding whether to follow the doctor's advice, patients may attach unwarranted importance to his or her bedside manners. Psychologists have labeled this phenomenon the *halo effect*, and found it in a number of situations. "If we think a baseball pitcher is handsome and athletic, for example, we are likely to rate him better at throwing the ball, too" (Kahneman 2011, p. 199). Patients, in other words, should learn to *distrust their trust*, just as doctors should learn to distrust their beliefs in their own competence and be willing to admit ignorance (see below).

Second, there may be *excusable ignorance* on the patient's part. As Dr. Reach mentions, if the doctor fails to educate the patient, he or she may pay excessive attention to the list of scary secondary effects – most of them very rare – that are usually listed on the instruction sheet that comes with the medication. In a very different set of cases, the patient may be exposed to a biased sample. People on dialysis sometimes refuse an offer to get a transplantation because the only transplantees they meet at the dialysis center are those whose grafts failed to take.

## Nonadherence by Doctors

Earlier, I mentioned why patient nonadherence could be rational, because of lack of trust in the doctor. The failure of doctors to adhere to recommendations can also be quite rational. In their case, the source of their nonadherence may not be lack of trust, but simply reflect their understanding of the limitations of recommendations generated by evidence-based medicine. As Dr. Reach notes, if the double-blind randomized trials that were the basis for recommending a given medication excluded older patients or patients with multiple pathologies, the doctor may in a given case well be justified in ignoring it. The well-informed doctor might also wonder whether the trial results might be biased because of nonadherence by subjects who suffered negative secondary effects. Also, nonadherence by the doctor may be rational in the face of the nonadherence on the part of the patients. Thus if a given level of some substance in the blood is not attained, the doctor may seek to improve the adherence of the patient rather than, as recommended by the guidelines, intensify the treatment.

Among the sources of irrational or unjustified nonadherence, Dr. Reach singles out, once again, myopia as a main culprit. In a phrase, *myopia causes inertia*, that is, under-treatment or non-treatment. Before I proceed, I want to mention the possibility of *overtreatment*, not, as in the case of my knee-surgery, because of the pecuniary interest of the doctor, but because of an engrained medical "tendency toward action rather than inaction". Such an error is more likely to happen with a doctor who is overconfident, whose ego is inflated, but it can also occur *when a physician is desperate and gives in to the urge to 'do something'*. The error, not infrequently, is sparked by pressure from a patient, and it takes considerable effort for a doctor to resist. 'Don't just do something, stand there', Dr. Linda Lewis, one of my mentors once said when I was unsure of a diagnosis". (Groopman 2007, p. 169; emphasis added). Even when the recommended procedure is to "wait and see", the doctor's *inaction-aversion* might get the better of him (see also Elster 2009).

Although doctors as well as patients are no doubt often subject to myopia, I suspect that in the case of doctors *uncertainty* as well as *blame-avoidance* may be more prominent causes of inertia. Few patients are so knowledgeable that they will blame their doctors for *not* prescribing a novel and recommended medication, but they might blame him if he does prescribe it and it turns out to have undesirable effects. Knowing this, the doctor may well stay with the status quo. From the doctor's personal point of view, risk-avoidance may not be irrational. If a recommended but risky operation fails and the patient brings suit for medical malpractice, the jury is very likely to be subject to *hindsight bias* and conclude that the doctor should have known that it was *too* risky (Sunstein et al. 2002). Anticipating this outcome, the doctor may decide that in the trade-off between the patient's expected health and his own expected income, the latter weighs more heavily. One may question the morality of his decision, but rationality and morality do not coincide, any more than do rationality and wisdom.

Let me conclude by citing two irrational sources of nonadherence by doctors to the official recommendations. The first, once again, is reactance. In an article cited by Dr. Reach, Dijsktra et al. (2000) show that "resistance to imposed activities (cookbook medicine)" is an important barrier to the implementation of diabetes guidelines in the Netherlands. The second and probably related source is the doctor's exaggerated belief in his or her clinical competence. Experts in a number of domains claim that their experience makes them sensitive to tell-tale signs that designers of a controlled study might ignore. Moreover, when different pieces of evidence point in different directions, experts claim to be able to draw on their experience to decide which, in any given case, should be given most weight. However, this favorable self-image, induced by the amour-propre of the doctors, is demonstrably false. Almost without exception, a simple mechanical formula based on a few variables will outperform the diagnoses and prognoses of experts, including doctors (Dawes et al. 1989).

## Conclusion

In the present book and in its companion volume, Dr. Reach brings out with unprecedented clarity and synthetic skills the realities of the medical universe. It may not surprise us that patients can be irrational, either when not complying with the doctor's prescriptions or complying when they should have questioned the advice. They are, after all, often in a highly stressful situation where normal critical faculties and decision-making capacity can be suspended. Groping after straws, terminal cancer patients often ignore the evidence-based advice of the oncologist and turn instead to a quack. By contrast, we would expect doctors to be calm, detached, and rational in their role as mediators between the medical authorities and the patients, disregarding recommendations when and only when they have adequate reasons for doing so. Unlike the patient, they have nothing at stake. As Dr. Reach shows, however, this idyllicizing picture is inaccurate. The amour-propre of doctors is at stake, and so is their professional reputation. Also, like the rest of us, doctors are subject to the *horror vacui*: "Many of this world's abuses are engendered – or to put it more rashly, all of this world's abuses are engendered – by our being schooled to be afraid to admit our ignorance and because we are required to accept anything which we cannot refute" (Montaigne 1991, p. 1159).

Jon Elster
Columbia University

## References

Ainslie G. Picoeconomics. Cambridge: Cambridge University Press; 1992.

Dawes R, Faust D, Meehl P. Clinical versus actuarial judgment. Science. 1989;243:1668–74.

Dijkstra R, Braspenning J, Uiters E, van Ballegooie E, Grol RT. Perceived barriers to the implementation of diabetes guidelines in hospitals in the Netherlands. Neth J Med. 2000;56:80–5.

Elster J. Explaining social behavior. Cambridge/New York: Cambridge University Press; 2007.

Elster J. Urgency. Inquiry. 2009;52:399–422.

Groopman B. How doctors think. Boston: Houghton-Mifflin; 2007.

Kahneman D. Thinking fast and slow. New York: Farrar, Straus and Giroux; 2011.

Lacan J. Écrits. Paris: Seuil; 1977.

Loewenstein G. Hot–cold empathy gaps and medical decision making. Health Psychol. 2005;24:S49–56.

Montaigne M de. Essays. London: Allen Lane; 1911.

Sunstein CR, Hastie R, Payne JW, Schkade DA, Viscu WK. Punitive damages, how juries decide. Chicago: University of Chicago Press; 2002.

# Foreword to the French Edition

It is not surprising that an experienced diabetologist, author of a book of reflection on patient adherence, turns to a hypertension specialist to draft an introduction on what is clinical inertia.

Being at the same time diseases and cardiovascular risk factors, hypertension and type 2 diabetes live together since 1970. At that time, indeed, the performance of a randomized clinical trial concluded that there are cardiovascular benefits to the treatment of hypertension [1], whereas the same technique applied to diabetes care instead drew attention to the risks derived from certain treatments [2]. From 1970 to 1990, the discovery of new anti-hypertensive therapeutic classes multiplied. This led each time to new clinical trials, whose meta-analysis establishes, without ambiguity, that independently of the class of medication used, a pharmacological reduction in blood pressure reproduces the benefits expected from observational studies on cardiovascular and renal mortality in its various components, and even on total mortality. Though the path was the same regarding the prevention of diabetic microangiopathy, the prevention of coronary events and strokes by the pharmacological reduction in blood glucose, and in its integrator $HbA_1C$, proved disappointing, glitazones included. Diabetes care, awaiting proof, benefits from new therapeutic classes which provide hope, beyond metformin and sulfonylureas [3, 4].

For both diseases, or risk factors, the multiplicity of results and the exponential growth of knowledge led the medical world to organize itself in groups of experts who regularly produce recommendations. The solemnity of this term is appreciated more by the administrators of the health care system than its relativity is perceived by those to whom they address. And the health care world wonders: why is it that what is demonstrated does not find itself entirely in care practices? Why aren't the results demonstrated by randomized clinical trials confirmed a hundred percent in populations? Is it a social phenomenon, linked to disparities of all kinds and all places, which makes it impossible, in the medical domain as in others, to establish an ideal world? Or should one look at the personal responsibility of those for whom the recommendations should provide, if they are patients, a brighter future, and if they are health care providers, a practice without reproach?

The second explanation seems more encouraging, and those who want to make the quality of long-term care progress concentrate their attention here. The discord between theoretically possible and desirable results and those obtained in current practice implies numerous responsibilities. They fall roughly into three areas. (1) The health care system in general, its imperfect organization, its limited accessibility. (2) The people with a disease and their lack of adherence. (3) The health care providers and their inertia. The term is new, dating a little more than ten years, and translates a lack of reactivity of medical decisions faced with a diagnostic or care situation which is nevertheless well codified [5]. The doctor sees the imperfection of results without reacting. The French term of "observance" is over forty years old, when the inappropriate English word of "compliance" was replaced by the appropriate name of "observance". Though necessary, the word compliance, useful in hemodynamics, has still unfortunately not been completely left behind, and the word still sometimes reappears. Those who worked on chronic inflammatory rheumatism and hypertension had chosen the word of observance to express the concordance between patient behavior and doctor prescriptions, with a touch of religious rule which translated the physician-patient relationship such as it was conceived and wished at the beginning of the 1970s.

Therefore it is logical that a hypertension specialist can be invited to introduce a diabetologist's book, and there is a logic of thought that this diabetologist extended his initial reflection on patients' adherence by an analysis of doctors' inertia.

In a first analysis, the lack of adherence can be felt as disobedience by patients, and the inertia of doctors as lack of conscientiousness and a superficiality of their practices. I'm doing what you prescribed, says the patient, without following the entire diet and without always taking all medications. I'm doing enough for you, says the doctor to her patient, without modifying a treatment which is working poorly, or even not at all. According to this mode of reasoning, it is necessary to obtain a "confession" of her nonadherence from the patient, to make her correct it (no, doctor, I did not take your …, it gives me a stomach ache. Impossible, take it or I cannot make you better…) In the same way, one must just as rationally denounce inertia (it's not perfect, but it's better than nothing, says the doctor, and the common sense of both partners makes them prefer the probability of not having the disease which one wants to prevent over the complexity of the prescription and the risk of the treatment …)

Officially, awareness of patient nonadherence and its multiple components – a first book – and awareness of medical inertia and its mechanisms beyond those of simple ignorance – another book – lead Dr. Reach to confide us his secret thoughts. Can one resist? Can nonadherence be considered as the normality of a person whom the medical intrusion disturbs, and who has the right to flee, even if, in addition to lack of respect for the doctor one should consider the cost to the health care system? Morality, or immorality? [6].

Likewise, can medical inertia translate a distrust of the "rule of the hour", and the norm? In a medicine defined by norms, is the justification of these norms sufficient to transform them into a quality requirement? In reality, the norm arises from clinical trials performed on volunteer people by volunteer health care providers, and their external validity is unreliable because 90 % of the people on whom the treatments are applied are not included in the scientific studies, generally due to a social, psychological or medical complexity. The lower the better, it is said, for blood pressure, glycated hemoglobin, or cholesterol levels, generally based on observational studies associated with randomized clinical trials [4, 7, 8]. But in daily life, age is associated with multiple pathologies, prescriptions become longer, psychology includes distrust and doubt [9].

Professor Reach's book will illuminate the complexity of human behavior. It will decrease nonadherence, it will fight inertia. The part which persists will be reduced so that rules are better applied, but between rules and medical error, will persist a grey area, shrunk little by little, a bit less dark, but the trace of an apparent common sense which one must know to distrust and of a part of humanism which one must cultivate …[10].

Joël Ménard
Paris 6 University

## References

1. Veterans Administration Cooperative Study Group on antihypertensive agents. Effects of treatment on morbidity in hypertension. Results in patients with diastolic blood pressure averaging 90 through 114 mmHg. JAMA. 1970;213:1143–52.
2. Goldner MG, Knatterud GL, Prout TE. Effects of hypoglycemic agents on vascular complications in patients with adult-onset diabetes. 3. Clinical implications of UGDP results. JAMA. 1971;218:1400–10.
3. Holman RR, Paul SK, Bethel MA, Matthews DR, Neil HA. 10-year follow-up of intensive glucose control in type 2 diabetes. N Engl J Med. 2008;359:1577–89.
4. Zoungas S, de Galan BE, Ninomiya T, Grobbee D, Hamet P, Heller S, MacMahon S, Marre M, Neal B, Patel A, Woodward M, Chalmers J. ADVANCE Collaborative Group. Cass A, Glasziou P, Harrap S, Lisheng L, Mancia G, Pillaj A, Poulter N, Perkovic V, Travert F. Combined effects of routine blood pressure lowering and intensive glucose control on macrovascular and microvascular outcomes in patients with type 2 diabetes: New results from the ADVANCE trial. N Engl J Med. 2011;364:818–28.
5. Phillips LS, Branch WT, Cook CB, Doyle JP, El-Kebbi IM, Gallina DL, Miller CD, Ziemer DC, Barnes CS. Clinical inertia. Ann Intern Med. 2001;135:825–34.
6. Reach G. Pourquoi se soigne-t-on, Enquête sur la rationalité morale de l'observance, Le Bord de L'Eau, 2007.
7. ACCORD Study Group, Gerstein HC, Miller ME, Genuth S, Ismail-Beigi F, Buse JB, Goff DC Jr, Probstfield JL, Cushman WC, Ginsberg HN, Bigger JT, Grimm RH Jr, Byington RP, Rosenberg YD, Friedewald WT. Long-term effects of intensive glucose lowering on cardiovascular outcomes. Diabetes Care. 2009;32:2068–74.
8. Law MR, Morris JK, Wald NJ. Use of blood pressure lowering drugs in the prevention of cardiovascular disease: meta-analysis of cardiovascular disease: 147 randomised trials in the context of expectations from prospective epidemiological studies. BMJ. 2009;338:b1665. doi:10.1136/bmj.b1665.
9. Zoungas S, Chalmers J, Ninomiya T, Li Q, Cooper ME, Colagiuri S, Fulcher G, de Galan BE, Harrap S, Hamet P, Heller S, MacMahon D, Marre M, Poulter N, Travert F, Patel A, Neal B, Woodward M; for the ADVANCE Collaborative Group. Association of HbA(1c) levels with vascular complications and death in patients with type 2 diabetes: evidence of glycaemic thresholds. Diabetologia. 2012;55:636–43.
10. Crowley MJ, Smith VA, Olsen MK, Danus S, Oddone EZ, Bosworth HB, Powers BJ. Treatment intensification in a hypertension telemanagement trial: clinical inertia or good clinical judgment? Hypertension. 2011;58:552–8.

# Contents

**1 Introduction** ....................................................... 1
  Four Perspectives ...................................................... 3
  References ............................................................ 3

**2 Definitions** ........................................................ 5
  Clinical Inertia ...................................................... 5
  Therapeutic Inertia and Clinical Inertia .............................. 6
  Clinical Practice Guidelines .......................................... 6
  Evidence-Based Medicine ............................................... 7
  Evidence Practice Gap ................................................. 7
  Medical Error ......................................................... 8
  What Is Not Clinical Inertia .......................................... 9
  Formal Definition of Clinical Inertia ................................. 10
    Definition: Physician Behavior Falls Under Clinical Inertia
    If and Only If ...................................................... 10
  References ............................................................ 11

**3 The Evidence: The Gap Between Guidelines and Clinical Reality** .... 13
  Introduction: Highlighting the Existence of the Phenomenon
  and Its Consequences .................................................. 13
    Consequences of Clinical Inertia .................................... 15
  Analysis of Clinical Inertia in Different Diseases .................... 17
    Diabetes ............................................................ 17
    Hypertension ........................................................ 20
    Hyperlipidemia ...................................................... 21
    Cardiovascular Risk Prevention ...................................... 21
    Other Conditions Where One Can Highlight
    the Clinical Inertia Phenomenon ..................................... 22
  References ............................................................ 25

**4 Determinants and Explanatory Models of Clinical Inertia** ......... 31
  Determinants of Clinical Inertia ...................................... 32
    Initial Explanations: Denial, Exaggerated Use of "Soft Reasons"
    and Physician Lack of Training on the Principle of Titration ........ 32
    Competing Demands ................................................... 32

xix

| | |
|---|---|
| The Effect of Uncertainty | 33 |
| Poor Appreciation of the Actual Situation of the Patient | 33 |
| Characteristics of the Physician | 34 |
| The Effect of Belonging to an Ethnic Minority and Being Disadvantaged | 34 |
| The Doctor, Her Patient and the Health Care System | 35 |
| Physician Clinical Inertia and Patient Nonadherence | 35 |
| Theoretical Explanatory Models of Clinical Inertia | 36 |
| The Knowledge-Attitude-Behavior-Result Model | 36 |
| The Awareness-Agreement-Adoption-Adherence Model | 38 |
| A Symmetrical Model Involving Physician and Patient: The Management of Dyslipidemia in Women | 39 |
| Physician Guideline Compliance Model | 39 |
| Another Psychological Model Applied to Comprehension of Clinical Inertia: The Regulatory Focus Theory | 40 |
| References | 42 |

**5 The Physician and Evidence-Based Medicine** ..................... 45

| | |
|---|---|
| A New Way to Practice Medicine | 45 |
| Objectives of Evidence-Based Medicine | 46 |
| Data and Guidelines: Different Levels of Evidence | 46 |
| What Is Not Evidence-Based Medicine | 47 |
| Evidence-Based Medicine: Clinical Practice Assisted by the Development of Clinical Practice Guidelines | 48 |
| Evidence-Based Medicine, Medicine Practiced Within a Context of Uncertainty | 50 |
| Evidence-Based Medicine: A Change of Paradigm? | 56 |
| Schrödinger's Cat and Einstein's Boxes | 58 |
| A Critique of Evidence-Based Medicine | 59 |
| The Physician Faced with a New Medicine | 59 |
| Theoretical Critiques of Evidence-Based Medicine | 60 |
| Epistemological Critique of the Concept of Evidence-Based Medicine | 64 |
| From an Evidence-Based Medicine to a Practice-Based Medicine | 65 |
| By Way of Provisional Conclusion: Guidelines or "Mindlines"? | 66 |
| References | 68 |

**6 To Do or Not to Do: A Critique of Medical Reason** ............... 73

| | |
|---|---|
| Definition | 73 |
| The Context of Uncertainty Which Surrounds All Medical Activities, and the Concept of Risk | 75 |
| The Notion of Heuristics and Bias | 76 |
| Different Heuristics Used in Human Judgment Within a Context of Uncertainty | 76 |

Contents xxi

Sources of Bias in Decisions Under Risk ......................... 78
Heuristics Are Necessary and Do Not Necessarily Have
an Adverse Effect............................................. 80
Heuristics, Principles of Evidence-Based Medicine,
and Medical Behavior: Coming Back to Clinical Inertia.............. 80
Role of Emotions in Medical Decisions ......................... 82
Emotions in Mental Life.................................... 82
Emotions in Medical Decisions ............................. 83
Emotions and Cognition: Two Components of Reason.............. 84
Emotions as Notification of the Feeling of Risk................. 84
Relationship Between Emotions and Behavior:
Rather Than Causation, a Feedback Dynamic ................... 86
Chagrin and Regret: Application to the Issue of Clinical Inertia ..... 87
Emotions in the Interaction Between Physician and Patient,
and in the Relationship Between Clinical Inertia and Nonadherence. . . 89
...Or Not to Do: Psychology of the Status Quo
and the Difficulty of Making a Decision ......................... 91
References ................................................... 93

**7  Overcoming *True* Clinical Inertia.** ............................. 97
Education................................................... 98
Initial Training of Physicians ............................... 98
Continuing Medical Education .............................. 99
Role of "Opinion Leaders" ................................. 100
Reminder and Feedback Systems ............................ 100
Facilitators ................................................. 102
Simplify Treatments, Use Treatments Having Fewer Side Effects.... 102
Overcoming Decisional Uncertainty Through Protocols .......... 102
Organizational Aspects .................................... 103
Reinforcement .............................................. 105
Incentive by Public Authorities: Pay for Performance ............ 105
Incentive by Patients...................................... 107
Incentive by Others: Peers, Pharmacists and Nurses ............. 108
Physician Self-Incentive: An Explanation Through
Philosophy of Mind........................................ 108
Force of Habit .............................................. 109
Can One Avoid Cognitive Biases?.............................. 110
Emotional Reversal: Using Emotions to Overcome Clinical Inertia..... 111
Concern: The Philosophical Dimension of Care.................. 112
Implementing Positive Emotions: Emotional Reversal............ 112
Physician Optimism and Pessimism .......................... 113
Trust, Pride and Self-Approval .............................. 113
References .................................................. 115

| 8 | **Conclusion: Time for Medical Reason** | 121 |
|---|---|---|
| | The Difference Between Two Dynamics | 123 |
| | Variability and Uncertainty | 124 |
| | What to Do with Emotions?. | 125 |
| | An Epistemological Transition: What the Phenomena of Physician Clinical Inertia and Patient Nonadherence Reveal | 126 |
| | Evidence-Based Medicine and Person-Centered Medicine | 128 |
| | Educational Value of Guidelines | 128 |
| | Tacit Nature of Knowledge and Holistic Base of "Mindlines" | 130 |
| | Appropriate Inaction and "True" Clinical Inertia: In Both Cases, Actions. | 131 |
| | Overcoming True Clinical Inertia | 132 |
| | Time for Medical Reason. | 133 |
| | References | 134 |

**By the Same Author** ......... 137

**Index** ......... 139

# Introduction

**1**

**Abstract**

Clinical Inertia is when a physician does not begin or intensify a treatment when this is deemed necessary according to current clinical practice guidelines. The term was coined in 2001 by Phillips et al. in an article appearing in the Annals of Internal Medicine. Initially described in diseases such as diabetes, hypertension and hypercholesterolemia, the concept spread to numerous chronic diseases. The purpose of this book is to offer, for the first time in English, a review of the data from the literature in this domain and to propose an explanation of this phenomenon which represents a major public health problem. This explanation uses a critical analysis first of the very nature of Evidence-Based Medicine from which guidelines stem and second of the psychological processes which preside over medical decisions, which are described here under the name of "medical reason" and of which this book proposes a "critique".

In the past, the purpose of medicine was essentially to relieve symptoms and to occasionally cure diseases. For about the past forty years, it also, and perhaps primarily, takes care of the treatment of chronic, often asymptomatic diseases, whose only initial manifestation is at times an abnormal reading: this is the case for example for diabetes, hypertension, hypercholesterolemia, where it's a matter of preventing long term deleterious consequences. In particular, treatment of some of these anomalies, which contribute to cardiovascular risk, provides an increased life expectancy. Indeed, effective drug treatments were developed and assessed, especially in terms of morbidity and mortality, in large clinical trials that form the corpus of what is commonly known as "Evidence-Based Medicine". Based on this *evidence*, "clinical practice guidelines" were developed and widely disseminated by Learned Societies and official institutions, such as, in France, the *Haute Autorité de Santé*.

In an ideal world, the advent of effective treatments and the clarification of their implementation through these guidelines should lead to a substantial improvement

© Springer International Publishing Switzerland 2015
G. Reach, *Clinical Inertia: A Critique of Medical Reason*,
DOI 10.1007/978-3-319-09882-1_1

in the percentage of patients whose abnormal reading is corrected or in whom the disease is controlled, therefore to the effective prevention of complications from chronic diseases and, thus, to an improvement in life expectancy of afflicted patients.

In 2001, one could make the following observations: blood pressure readings were corrected in only 45 % of patients treated for hypertension, the recommended target of 7 % glycated hemoglobin was reached in only 33 % of diabetic patients treated, and LDL-cholesterol was within the guidelines' target in only 14–38 % of patients, depending on the study. Of course, this could be due to the difficulty, within a given disease, of obtaining "normal readings"; or else, one could blame therapeutic failures on the nonadherence of patients who do not take their prescribed medication. Nevertheless, another barrier to the efficiency of care has emerged: in fact, only 53 % of hypertensive patients, 17–23 % of patients with hypercholesterol-emia, and 73 % of diabetic patients, *in whom the disease was known, were treated*. These *anomalies* were but the illustration of a gap, whose existence had begun to be recognized over the past twenty years: that between guidelines coming from clinical trials and clinical practice in its daily reality, often referred to as "real life".

This analysis led Lawrence Phillips to propose that lack of treatment implementation or intensification until the target has been reached, in compliance with current guidelines, could represent a major obstacle to the effective management of chronic diseases. He gave a name to this phenomenon: *Clinical Inertia* [1].

Let's consider as example a diabetic patient treated in the year 2000 with oral antidiabetic agents at maximum dose, whose HbA1c glycated hemoglobin level (for example 9.2 %) is not within target, who has lost weight and does not appear to be deviating from her diet. According to the current guidelines at the time, insulin therapy is clearly indicated. The patient is resistant to this idea, for a variety of reasons, which one can understand. Yet this *psychological insulin resistance* [2] also afflicts her physician, who shies away from the decision, puts it off till the next appointment and does not even offer the patient insulin, thus demonstrating clinical inertia: it seems that "patients and physicians have often colluded in implicit and unspoken contracts to continue oral agents for as long as possible", as one can read in an article whose very title suggests that treatment failure is due to a "conspiracy" between the disease, suboptimal therapy, but also patient and physician attitudes [3].

But such an *attitude* on the part of the physician is not limited to the shift to an injectable treatment. Clinical inertia can also manifest itself through lack of treatment intensification in the form of either a dose increase of medications already prescribed or the prescription of "one more medication", what one calls "titration" of treatment. And, as we have seen, sometimes diagnosed diseases are simply not treated: when we begin to assess the *actual* implementation of care, we see that we do not always do what we should do, undoubtedly with reasons: *I'll do it the next time, perhaps this will get better on its own, perhaps better patient adherence to her treatment and diet, and more physical activity will allow me to avoid treatment intensification* [4] or else, *today there is a more urgent problem to resolve, and besides, today's elevated blood pressure reading might be due to the white coat effect etc.*

Thus, it seems like these attitudes of health care provider clinical inertia and patient nonadherence can be considered as the two faces of a Janus who opposes the efficiency of care. They represent in fact the major discrepancy between that which can be demonstrated in a clinical trial and "real life": in clinical trials (which, as we have seen, served to forge Evidence-Based Medicine from which come clinical practice guidelines), patients are generally adherent and physicians are guided by a protocol in order to not be inert. But in real life, it is up to the physician alone to apply the guideline to *this* patient she is faced with, and, it is up to *this* patient to follow the physician's prescription.

Regarding patient nonadherence, in 2003 the WHO declared that increasing the effectiveness of adherence interventions may have a far greater impact on the health of the population than any improvement in specific medical treatments – since a medication that is prescribed but not taken, is ineffective [5]. The same may well be true of the phenomenon of clinical inertia: if guidelines are not applied, it could happen, for example, that a treatment which could have been effective is not prescribed. The two phenomena of nonadherence and inertia thus have consequences, not only for the sick individual, but also in terms of health care expenditure, and therefore for society [6].

## Four Perspectives

The purpose of this book is first to present the epidemiological data available on clinical inertia which will demonstrate the breadth of the phenomenon and its consequences; then, to analyze its mechanisms. Its objective is to show how individual behavior leads to the emergence of a major public health problem which health care systems are attempting to tackle through different means. This is therefore both an *epidemiological* and *psychological* study of the clinical inertia phenomenon.

It may seem at first glance surprising that physicians conduct themselves in an "inert" manner with their patients, just as one can be surprised by patient nonadherence: how, simply, is all this possible? To ask if something is *possible* is a typically *philosophical* question: unlike psychologists who ask *how* things can happen, philosophers are interested in the conceptual framework which separates the possible from the impossible [7]. But the question asked by the existence of phenomena such as physician clinical inertia or patient nonadherence also has a fundamentally *epistemological* nature: it forces us to reconsider in the era of Evidence-Based Medicine not only the human factor in medical practice, but also in fact the very foundations of this new, *rationalized*, way to practice medicine: it leads thus to a critical analysis of what we can call *medical reason*.

## References

1. Phillips LS, Branch WT, Cook CB, Doyle JP, El-Kebbi IM, Gallina DL, Miller CD, Ziemer DC, Barnes CS. Clinical inertia. Ann Intern Med. 2001;135:825–34.
2. Leslie CA, Satin-Rapaport W, Matheson D, Stone R, Enfield G. Psychological insulin resistance: a missed diagnosis. Diabetes Spectr. 1994;7:52–7.

3. Wallace TM, Matthews DR. Poor glycaemic control in type 2 diabetes: a conspiracy of disease, suboptimal therapy and attitude. Q J Med. 2000;93:369–74.
4. Branch WT, Higgins S. Clinical inertia: hard to move it forward. Rev Esp Cardiol. 2010; 63:1399–401.
5. WHO. Adherence to long term therapies, evidence for action. Geneva: World Health Organization Publications; 2003.
6. Scheen AJ. Inertie thérapeutique dans la pratique médicale: causes, conséquences, solutions. Rev Med Liège. 2010;65:232–38.
7. Pears D. Motivated irrationality. South Bend: St Augustine's Press; 1998. p. 1.

# Definitions

**2**

## Abstract

In this chapter, we define the following terms: clinical inertia, therapeutic inertia, clinical practice guidelines, Evidence-Based Medicine, evidence practice gap, and medical error. In particular, we insist straightaway on the fact that lack of treatment intensification is not always a case of clinical inertia, but can represent on the contrary a carefully thought out decision on the part of the physician. This incites one to think about the quality criteria which preside over the evaluation of the quality of medical behaviors. At the end of the chapter, we propose a formal definition of true clinical inertia: physician behavior falls under Clinical Inertia *if and only if*

1. a Guideline (G) exists, explicit or implicit
2. the doctor (D) knows the Guideline (G)
3. the doctor (D) thinks that this Guideline (G) applies to the patient (P)
4. the doctor (D) has the resources to apply the Guideline (G)
5. conditions 1–4 have been met, yet the doctor (D) does not follow the Guideline (G) in the case of the patient (P).

## Clinical Inertia

Historically speaking, one should pay justice to Cabana et al. [1] for having not only formally recognized the existence of the phenomenon – "Despite wide promulgation, clinical practice guidelines have had limited effect on changing physician behavior" – but especially for having understood that it could be fruitful to analyze its causes: "Physician adherence to guidelines may be hindered by a variety of barriers. A theoretical approach can help explain these barriers and possibly help target interventions to specific barriers."

The term *clinical inertia* appears to have been used for the first time that same year by Lawrence Phillips' team in Atlanta in the title of an article showing that it is possible to improve diabetes control by "overcoming clinical inertia" of health care

© Springer International Publishing Switzerland 2015
G. Reach, *Clinical Inertia: A Critique of Medical Reason*,
DOI 10.1007/978-3-319-09882-1_2

providers [2]; but it was officially established in 2001 in the seminal article by Phillips et al., entitled *Clinical Inertia*, published in the *Annals of Internal Medicine*, with the following definition [3]: "The goals for management are well defined, effective therapies are widely available, and practice guidelines for each of these diseases have been disseminated extensively. Despite such advances, health care providers often do not initiate or intensify therapy appropriately during visits of patients with these problems. *We define such behavior as clinical inertia— recognition of the problem, but failure to act.*"

## Therapeutic Inertia and Clinical Inertia

The term *therapeutic inertia* was used for the first time in the medical literature in 2004 by Andrade et al. [4] regarding drug treatment of hypertension and was taken up by Okonofua et al. [5] who defined therapeutic inertia as "the providers' failure to increase therapy when treatment goals are unmet [...], begin new medications or increase dosages of existing medications when an abnormal clinical parameter is recorded".

One sees that the two definitions are in fact very close: these two articles on therapeutic inertia essentially concerned the study of drug-taking but, when the problem is considered more globally, the use of the terms clinical inertia and therapeutic inertia appears interchangeable. Thus, Allen et al. [6] proposed to regroup under the term *clinical inertia* the different aspects covering the underutilization of therapies recognized as effective, with an adequate or even overwhelming level of proof, in preventing the occurrence of different clinical events such as death, nonfatal myocardial infarction, or stroke. For Allen, these different aspects entail not only obstacles to care coming from the physician and the health care system, but also from the patient (her nonadherence), thus adopting an analysis proposed by O'Connor et al. in 2005 [7]. This has the value of showing the link between the two phenomena of health care provider clinical inertia – a noncompliance with current guidelines – and of patient nonadherence with recommendations from her physician.

One can note that patient nonadherence, for its part, concerns all aspects of treatment: not only prescribed medication and self-monitoring, but also changes in lifestyle, advice regarding tobacco, alcohol, the carrying out prescribed lab tests, showing up for appointments etc. [8]. The same is true of clinical inertia: clinical practice guidelines do not concern only drug-taking, but also prescription of lifestyle measures, monitoring and the frequency of appointments, the carrying out of screening tests, even the practice of patient education in chronic diseases, and each of these aspects can be lacking in patient management. Thus, in diabetes care, lack of multiannual HbA1c monitoring or annual prescription of a dilated eye examination or microalbumin urine test, even foot monitoring in patients at risk can fall within clinical inertia.

## Clinical Practice Guidelines

These are "systematically developed statements to assist practitioner and patient decisions about appropriate health care for specific clinical circumstances" [9, 10]. The goal is to inform health care professionals, but also patients (in France, the guidelines developed by the *Haute Autorité de Santé* are accessible online without restriction) on the state of the art and the data acquired from science in order to improve management and quality of care. Their implementation is expected to decrease the variability in therapeutic management from one case to another and to accelerate the application of progress considered as effective into daily practice [9].

## Evidence-Based Medicine

It's in 1992 that this term was used for the first time by Guyatt et al. [11] in an article considered as the culmination of a school of thought initiated 20 years earlier by Cochrane [12] who wrote: "It is surely a great criticism of our profession that we have not organized a critical summary, by specialty or subspecialty, adapted periodically, of all relevant randomized controlled trials" [13].

This "new way" to practice medicine "integrates the best external evidence with individual clinical expertise and patient's choice." It is important, following this classic definition, to immediately specify the following point: the founders of this approach insist upon the fact that this is in no way a matter of proposing cookbook medicine [14]: "Because it requires a bottom up approach that integrates the best external evidence with individual clinical expertise and patients' choice, it cannot result in slavish, cookbook approaches to individual patient care."

This precision will be crucial in tackling the issue of clinical inertia. Indeed, whereas the phenomenon of patient nonadherence has been known since Hippocrates (even though the concept of compliance was introduced in medicine only in 1979) (see [8]), the existence of the phenomenon of clinical inertia was recognized, as we have seen, much more recently: in fact, one can only speak of clinical inertia in relation to the existence of guidelines (which are not followed). One can therefore say that the emergence of clinical inertia *or rather its recognition as a medical issue* is a consequence of the advent of Evidence-Based Medicine. Yet we will see that two essential elements allow us to explain the existence of the phenomenon of clinical inertia: first, the difference between, on the one side *the Evidence* that forms the corpus of this new medical approach and which was obtained based on observation of cohorts of patients, and, on the other side the individual nature of all medical decisions; second, *the uncertainty* which these decisions must deal with: one can recall here the famous aphorism by William Osler [15] – "medicine is a science of uncertainty and an art of probability."

In other words, perhaps there is "Evidence"; there cannot be "proof".

## Evidence Practice Gap

This term describes the difference between the current state of knowledge and what is in fact carried out in common practice [16, 17]. This may concern the performance of lab tests, therapeutic strategies (prescription or intensification of treatment), prescription of lifestyle changes (for example, dietary guidelines, advice on physical activity or quitting smoking).

Thus, the difficulty for physicians to change their behavior regarding clinical practice guidelines was reported as of 1987: Kosecoff et al. showed, regarding 12 guidelines on breast cancer treatment, the performance of cesarean sections or coronary bypass surgery that their publication had had almost no effect on the behavior of physicians working in 10 hospitals in the state of Washington [18]. Likewise, in 1989, though a guideline aiming to decrease the performance of cesarean sections had been published 3 years earlier in Canada, a study showed that obstetricians generally were aware of its existence and approved of it; but, an audit of practices revealed that the actual changes were considerably less significant than what was declared by practitioners [19]. Fifteen years later, a study in the United States again showed that patients received only 55 % of recommended care: to take but two examples, only 24 % of diabetic patients had had at least 3 HbA1c measurements over a period of 2 years, and only 45 % of patients who had had a myocardial infarction received beta-blockers [20].

One can give a recent example illustrating the difficulty of translating new *evidence* into medical behavior: in 2002, a randomized clinical study (Diabetes Prevention Project) clearly showed the value of implementation of lifestyle measures or treatment with metformin in patients with "pre-diabetes" (impaired fasting glucose or glucose intolerance), which in 2005 led the American Diabetes Association to recommend those treatments to these patients. A study published in the United States in 2010 on a representative sample of the American population of 1,547 non-diabetic adults, showed that 19.4 % had impaired fasting glucose, 5.4 % had glucose intolerance, and 9.8 % had both conditions. Yet none of these patients had received treatment with metformin and guidelines regarding physical activity or diet were given in only one third of cases. The authors did not resolve between the possibilities that physicians might not be aware of the *evidence*, or that they might not be convinced by it, or else that they demonstrate inertia [21]. Likewise, a French study carried out in a hospital setting analyzed the behavior of physicians regarding current guidelines, showing a delay in introducing drug treatment in diabetic patients treated by diet alone, and an underutilization of biguanides [22].

The data, which will be presented further in this book, regarding clinical inertia encountered in different chronic diseases, confirms the existence of this gap between guidelines and clinical practice, the existence of which was recognized before the term clinical inertia was even forged [23, 24]. At a population level, this gap obviously represents a major public health problem: the term chasm was also used to describe the phenomenon.

## Medical Error

The fact that *true clinical inertia*, whose deleterious consequences for the patient we will describe, represents a medical error is not immediately apparent. Indeed, when one thinks of medical errors, one thinks more of errors *of commission*, those *which one commits* – whose consequences constitute that which one defines under the term iatrogenic: one speaks of adverse effects, some of which are avoidable when they result from medical errors [25].

Yet in the case of clinical inertia, it is typically an error *of omission*, represented *by what one did not do*: *a failure to act*, stated Phillips et al. in their article [3]. Thus, shortly after Phillips' publication, a study aimed to describe the nature of different medical errors felt as such by family physicians (they were asked to describe deleterious events which should not have occurred and which made them think: "this should not happen in my practice, and I never want this to happen again"); clinical inertia – or a similar concept – was not mentioned as being part of the "taxonomy" of medical errors [26]. Since, two publications, in diabetes treatment, have clearly referred to behavior falling under clinical inertia as "medical errors" [27, 28].

## What Is Not Clinical Inertia

In the conclusion of their article, Phillips et al. insisted [3]: of course, to not begin a treatment or to not intensifying it, to "renew a prescription" when guidelines would propose to modify it, is at times justified and therefore does not necessarily fall under clinical inertia; it may be on the contrary a carefully thought out decision transmitting the clinical finesse of the practitioner: "Experienced clinicians will recognize that exceptions always occur and that rigid insistence on the uniform application of guidelines for patient management could result in overtreatment or inappropriate actions."

Incidentally, this implies that one must be cautious when using lack of treatment intensification as an index of inappropriate quality of care. Indeed, quality measurements in this field can be made on three levels. (1) One can, in a population at risk, quantify the occurrence of events (for example death, a stroke etc.). Nevertheless, these events are often rare (and even more and more rare, since patients are nevertheless better and better treated!), which requires studies of large populations; these are often late in coming, which requires long term studies; what's more, they often depend more on factors linked to the patients than the care which they've received. (2) One can focus on intermediate markers, for example control of blood pressure levels which has been shown to be associated with the subsequent occurrence of events such as a stroke. Nevertheless, these intermediate markers, likewise, depend on factors coming as much from patients as from medical interventions. (3) One understands therefore that most quality measurements concern medical practices themselves – which brings us back to the issue of clinical inertia: for example, is blood pressure measured and a foot examination conducted at each appointment in diabetic patients? Was statin prescribed in compliance with current guidelines? But here also, on the one hand one must be sure that these criteria are associated with a decrease in the rate of pathological events, which is the goal of the management of chronic diseases. On the other hand, one must be able to take into account the exceptions which justify lack of implementation of the criterion considered [29].

This last crucial point, should invite one on the one hand to avoid assessing the "performance" of a physician based on an intermediate criterion, and on the other hand to nuance the diagnosis of clinical inertia. This was clearly highlighted in a study specifically on the management of hypercholesterolemia: it showed that in a population of 1,154 diabetic patients, in which 27 % of patients had elevated LDL-cholesterol above 130 mg/dl, in only 13 % of cases could treatment be considered inappropriate. Indeed, among the other 15 % of cases (159 patients), 117 had in fact actually received statin, or else the medication dose had been increased within the last 6 months, 8 already had the maximum dose of the medication, 12 had had a new measure showing a reading below 130 mg/dl, and 22 patients had a contraindication to the treatment [30]. Likewise, a study of treatment intensification in hypertensive patients revealed that very often lack of treatment modification took into account the patient's age, comorbidities, the polypharmacy already taken by the patient, and possible side effects of medications, and could therefore be justified [31].

It is therefore better in these cases to speak of *inaction*, rather than inertia. Thus, in an empirical study, two panels of physicians were questioned on the reasons which could lead them to not intensify a treatment. Based on these surveys, the authors constructed a model suggesting that about 60 % of reasons to not intensify treatment considered as significant (for example patient nonadherence or the white coat effect) could fall within *appropriate inaction* [32]. Another study even showed that the reasons given by physicians to no apply a guideline (the "exceptions") *were justified in 93 % of cases* when they were analyzed by peers [33].

## Formal Definition of Clinical Inertia

It is therefore necessary to give a strict definition of clinical inertia. We have proposed the following formal definition, which allows one at the same time to distinguish clinical inertia from situations where guidelines do not exist, from ignorance (the physician is not aware of guidelines which exist), appropriate inaction (she thinks the guideline does not apply to this patient here) or inertia linked to a lack of resources (no one can achieve the impossible) [34].

## Definition: Physician Behavior Falls Under Clinical Inertia If and Only If

1. a Guideline (G) exists, explicit or implicit
2. the doctor (D) knows the Guideline (G)
3. the doctor (D) thinks that this Guideline (G) applies to the patient (P)
4. the doctor (D) has the resources to apply the Guideline (G)
5. conditions 1–4 have been met, yet the doctor (D) does not follow the Guideline (G) in the case of the patient (P).

The merit of Phillips' publication which appears to have opened a true Pandora's Box, was to propose that such apparently *abnormal* situations, exist. The goal of this book is to try to understand how this is possible.

## References

1. Cabana MD, Rand CS, Powe NR, Wu AW, Wilson MH, Abboud P-A C, Rubin HR. Why don't physicians follow clinical practice guidelines? A framework for improvement. JAMA. 1999;282:1458–67.
2. Cook CB, Ziemer DC, El-Kebbi IM, Gallina DL, Dunbar VG, Ernst KL, Phillips LS. Diabetes in urban African-Americans. XVI. Overcoming clinical inertia improves glycemic control in patients with type 2 diabetes. Diabetes Care. 1999;22:1494–500.
3. Phillips LS, Branch WT, Cook CB, Doyle JP, El-Kebbi IM, Gallina DL, Miller CD, Ziemer DC, Barnes CS. Clinical inertia. Ann Intern Med. 2001;135:825–34.
4. Andrade SE, Gurwitz JH, Field TS, Kelleher M, Majumdar SR, Reed G, Black R. Hypertension management: the care gap between clinical guidelines and clinical practice. Am J Manag Care. 2004;10:481–6.
5. Okonofua EC, Simpson KN, Jesri A, Durkalski VL, Egan BM. Therapeutic inertia is an impediment to achieving the healthy people 2010 blood pressure control goals. Hypertension. 2006;47:345–51.
6. Allen JD, Curtiss FR, Fairman KA. Nonadherence, clinical inertia, or therapeutic inertia? J Manag Care Pharm. 2009;15:690–5.
7. O'Connor PJ, Sperl-Hillen JM, Johnson PE, Rush WA. Identification, classification, and frequency of medical errors in outpatient diabetes care. In: Henriksen K, Battles JB, Marks ES, Lewin DI, editors. Advances in patient safety: from research to implementation, vol 2: Concepts and methodology. Rockville: Agency for Healthcare Research and Quality (US); 2005.
8. Reach G. The mental mechanisms of patient adherence to long term therapies, mind and care, foreword by Pascal Engel, "Philosophy and Medicine" series, Springer, forthcoming.
9. Field MJ, Lohr KN, editors. Clinical practice guidelines: directions for a new program, institute of medicine. Washington, DC: National Academy Press; 1990.
10. HAS. Méthodes d'élaborations des recommandations de bonne pratique. http://www.has-sante.fr/portail/jcms/c_5233. Accessed 7 Apr 2014.
11. Evidence Based Medicine Working Group. Evidence-based medicine. A new approach to teaching the practice of medicine. JAMA. 1992;268:2420–5.
12. Cochrane AL. Effectiveness and efficiency: random reflections on health services. London: Nuffield Provincial Hospitals Trust; 1972 (réédition 1989, Royal Society of Medicine Press, London).
13. Cochrane AL. 1931–1971: a critical review, with particular reference to the medical profession. In: Medicines for the year 2000. London: Office of Health Economics; 1979. p. 1–11.
14. Sackett DL, Rosenberg WMC, Gray JAM, Haynes RB, Richardson WS. Evidence based medicine: what it is and what it isn't. BMJ. 1996;312:71–2.
15. Sir Osler W. The art, aphorism 265. Aphorisms from his bedside teachings and writings. Epitomes collected by Robert Bennett Bean, Charles C. Thomas, Springfield Ill, 1961.
16. Evidence-Practice Gaps. Complete report, vol 1. http://www.nhmrc.gov.au/_files_nhmrc/file/nics/material_resources/Evidence_volumeonecolour.pdf. Accessed 7 Apr 2014.
17. Liang L. The gap between evidence and practice. Health Aff. 2007;26:w119–21.
18. Kosecoff J, Kanouse DE, Rogers WH, McClosey L, Winslow CM, Brook RH. Effects of the national institutes of health consensus development program on physician practice. JAMA. 1987;258:2708–13.
19. Lomas J, Anderson GM, Domnick-Pierre K, Vayda E, Enkin MW, Hannah WJ. Do practice guidelines guide practice? The effect of a consensus statement on the practice of physicians. N Engl J Med. 1989;321:1306–11.
20. McGlynn EA, Asch SM, Adams J, Keesey J, Hicks J, DeCristofaro A, Kerr EA. The quality of health care delivered to adults in the United States. N Engl J Med. 2003;348:2635–45.
21. Karve A, Hayward RA. Prevalence, diagnosis, and treatment of impaired fasting glucose and impaired glucose tolerance in nondiabetic U.S. adults. Diabetes Care. 2010;33:2355–9.
22. Toussi M, Ebrahiminia V, Le Toumelin P, Cohen R, Venot A. An automated method for analyzing adherence to therapy guidelines: application in diabetes. In: Andersen SK et al., editors. E-Health beyond the horizon –get IT there. Amsterdam/Oxford: IOS Press; 2008. p. 339–44.

23. Davis DA, Taylor-Vaisey A. Translating guidelines into practice, a systematic review of theoretic concepts, practical experience and research evidence in the adoption of clinical practice guidelines. Can Med Assoc J. 1997;157:408–16.
24. Grimshaw JM, Thomas RE, MacLennan G, Fraser C, Ramsay CR, Vale L, Whitty P, Eccles MP, Matowe L, Shirran L, Wensing M, Dijkstra R, Donaldson C. Effectiveness and efficiency of guideline dissemination and implementation strategies. Executive summary. Health Technol Assess. 2004;8(6):iii–iv, 1–72.
25. Kohn LT, Corrigan JM, Donaldson MS. To err is human: building a safer health system, free executive summary. National Academy Press; 2000. http://www.nap.edu/catalog/9728.html. Accessed 7 Apr 2014.
26. Dovey SM, Meyers DS, Phillips Jr RL, Green LA, Fryer GE, Galliher JM, Kappus J, Grob P. A preliminary taxonomy of medical errors in family practice. Qual Saf Health Care. 2002;11:233–8.
27. Kennedy AG, MacLean CD. Clinical inertia: errors of omission in drug therapy. Am J Health Syst Pharm. 2004;61:401–4.
28. O'Connor PJ, Sperl-Hillen JAM, Johnson PE, Rush WA, Biltz G. Clinical inertia and outpatient medical errors. In: Henriksen K, Battles JB, Marks ES, Lewin DI, editors. Advances in patient safety: from research to implementation, vol 2: Concepts and methodology. Rockville: Agency for Healthcare Research and Quality (US); 2005.
29. Kerr EA, Krein SR, Vijan S, Hofer TP, Hayward RA. Avoiding pitfalls in chronic disease quality measurement: a case for the next generation of technical quality measures. Am J Manag Care. 2001;7:1033–43.
30. Kerr EA, Smith DM, Hogan MM, Hofer TP, Krein SR, Bermann M, Hayward RA. Building a better quality measure. Are some patients with "poor quality" actually getting good care? Med Care. 2003;41:1173–82.
31. Hicks PC, Westfall JM, Van Vorst RF, Bublitz Emsermann C, Dickinson LM, Pace W, Parnes B. Action or inaction? Decision making in patients with diabetes and elevated blood pressure in primary care. Diabetes Care. 2006;29:2580–5.
32. Safford MM, Shewchuk R, Qu H, Williams JH, Estrada CA, Ovalle F, Allison JJ. Reasons for not intensifying medications: differentiating "clinical inertia" from appropriate care. J Gen Intern Med. 2007;22:1648–55.
33. Persell SD, Dolan NC, Friesema EM, Thompson JA, Kaiser D, Baker DW. Frequency of inappropriate medical exceptions to quality measures. Ann Intern Med. 2010;152:225–31.
34. Reach G. Inertie clinique: comment est-elle possible? Médecine des Maladies Métaboliques. 2011;5:567–73.

# The Evidence: The Gap Between Guidelines and Clinical Reality

**3**

### Abstract

The phenomenon of clinical inertia represents a barrier to the efficiency of care in most chronic diseases. The purpose of this chapter is to review the recent literature, analyzing a hundred references, demonstrating the breadth of the phenomenon and its consequences, in particular in term of loss of chance for the patient: for example, lack of treatment intensification of diabetes or hypertension represents a cause of persistent disequilibrium which can have severe consequences on the appearance of complications of these diseases. This chapter analyzes in detail the data concerning clinical inertia in the following diseases: diabetes (a particular case of clinical inertia is the "psychological insulin resistance" of physicians who avoid prescription of insulin), hypertension, hyperlipidemia, cardiovascular risk, heart failure, cardiac valvular diseases, complete arrhythmia due to atrial fibrillation, asthma, osteoporosis, and gives bibliographical references concerning other diseases.

## Introduction: Highlighting the Existence of the Phenomenon and Its Consequences

A retrospective study [1] carried out in 2002–2003, on a population of over two million people covered by the Californian health insurance system Kaiser Permanente, in which close to 650,000 people had hypertension, dyslipidemia, or diabetes, made it possible to specify the percentage of patients that did not receive, 6 months after observation of insufficient control, treatment modification, and what occurred 6 months after that (Table 3.1).

Regarding hypertension, readings are in fact better than what was described in an older article assessing intensification of treatments in a cohort of 800 patients: within appointments where diastolic blood pressure was ≥90 mmHg, and systolic blood pressure ≥155 mmHg, treatment was intensified in only 25.6 % of cases. In

© Springer International Publishing Switzerland 2015
G. Reach, *Clinical Inertia: A Critique of Medical Reason*,
DOI 10.1007/978-3-319-09882-1_3

**Table 3.1** Highlighting of clinical inertia

|  | Hypertension (systolic) | Hypertension (diastolic) | Dyslipidemia (LDL-cholesterol) | Diabetes (HbA1c) |
|---|---|---|---|---|
| Number of uncontrolled patients |  |  |  |  |
|  | 125,427 | 31,121 | 132,266 | 48,568 |
| **Inappropriate care (no treatment modification)** |  |  |  |  |
|  | **28.8 %** | **17.6 %** | **41.4 %** | **30.3 %** |
| **Six months after** |  |  |  |  |
| Return to control | 7.7 % | 3.6 % | 6.2 % | 5.7 % |
| No return to control | 11.5 % | 5.3 % | 8.6 % | 7.3 % |
| No new measurement and no treatment modification | 9.6 % | 8.7 % | 26.6 % | 17.3 % |

Adapted from Rodondi et al. [1], Reproduced with permission of the American College of Physicians © 2006

this study, physicians did not appear to be ignoring elevated blood pressure readings since poorly controlled patients were seen 2–3 weeks earlier than those whose blood pressure was controlled [2].

The study by Okonofua et al., of 7,253 patients, followed by 168 physicians, with $6.4 \pm 0.03$ appointments within a year, made it possible to calculate more precisely a therapeutic inertia score, defined as the difference between the expected medication change rate (number of visits with elevated blood pressure/total number of visits) and the observed medication change rate (actual number of visits in which medications were increased/total number of visits). The therapeutic inertia score was $0.44 \pm 0.19$. In this study, a multivariate analysis specified the predictive factors of physician therapeutic inertia: the moderate nature of blood pressure readings, advanced age of the patient, low number of medications already prescribed, presence of coronary heart disease, of heart failure, copresence of diabetes and hypercholesterolemia [3].

In the field of diabetes, a recent French study examined 17,493 patients treated only with oral hypoglycemic agents with at least two available HbA1c measures, among which 3,118 (18 %) required treatment intensification according to current guidelines. Within these patients, only 39 % received such intensification in the 6 months following a second high measure (59 % at 12 months) [4]

In this study, the probability of treatment intensification was significantly positively associated with two factors: the younger the patient or the more her HbA1c level at the first available measure was elevated (up to a threshold of 9 %). Undoubtedly in many cases of "inaction" it was therefore appropriate, in accordance with recent data suggesting that in elderly patients, too great a treatment intensification can be dangerous. Another study, PANORAMA, also showed to what extent the reasons to not intensify treatment in the case of diabetes are complex, and that it is undoubtedly unjust to treat as inert behavior which is undoubtedly often appropriate [5].

Here also, these results appear to be in fact better than what was described in a previous American study, of 23,291 patients: even though HbA1c >8 % was found in 39 % of patients, treatment intensification took place in only 9.8 % of appointments [6].

Introduction: Highlighting the Existence of the Phenomenon and Its Consequences        15

In the field of hyperlipidemia, a study analyzed 5,028 appointments by 155 physicians [7]. In 73.6 % of cases, LDL-cholesterol was not controlled according to the current guidelines. Therapeutic inertia was observed in 42.8 % of these appointments. In 28.9 % of cases, the inertia was considered as "very high" since lack of treatment modification faced with LDL-cholesterol above 1.00 g/l was observed in patients with two other vascular risk factors (diabetes, smoking, hypertension).

Thus, retrospective studies, including those which have just been cited, can show the frequency of cases in which there appears to be a lack of treatment intensification. Nevertheless, this must be nuanced by what has already been mentioned: it is clear that "renewing the prescription" does not necessarily mean clinical inertia and that at least some of these cases can be justified. True clinical inertia is that where one cannot find such a justification. In the study by Kerr, this was the case for 113 among the 307 patients (or 37 % of cases) who had elevated LDL-cholesterol and whose treatment remained unchanged [8]. A recent study in the field of hypertension showed that physicians could not justify their decision in only about one third of cases [9].

## Consequences of Clinical Inertia

Yet a deleterious effect of lack of treatment intensification can be revealed.

Thus, regarding hypertension, Berlowitz showed that over a period of 2 years, systolic blood pressure decreased by 6.3 mmHg in patients having a more intensive treatment, and on the contrary increased by 4.8 mm in patients having a less intensive treatment [2]. More precisely, in the study by Okonofua [3], patients treated by physicians belonging to the least inert quintile (therapeutic inertia score = $0.10 \pm 0.002$) had a 32.7 times greater chance (95 % Confidence Interval: 25.1–42.6, $p < 0.0001$) of having their blood pressure controlled than those treated by physicians belonging to the most inert quintile of physicians (score = $0.73 \pm 0.002$). More recently, in the STITCH study, of 2,030 hypertensive patients, among which 42 % had blood pressure that was uncontrolled through treatment, a multivariate analysis showed that titration of treatment (increase in dose or number of medications) was an independent predictive factor of decrease in blood pressure [10].

Does decreasing physician clinical inertia improve blood pressure readings? The answer to this question is mixed: a positive effect was observed in certain studies [11–14], but not in a recent randomized intervention study where blood pressure readings remained unchanged, even though clinical inertia itself was indeed decreased [15].

Nevertheless, a study showed that physicians, when they do not intensify treatment in response to a computer alert informing them that a patient's blood pressure is elevated, are perhaps right when they give as argument the fact that the blood pressure readings were in fact moderately elevated: indeed, a retrospective analysis of blood pressure readings shows that they were less elevated in these cases than when physicians decided to intensify treatment; especially, in the months following, there were less often alerts of elevated readings in patients for whom treatment had not been intensified, which suggests that lack of treatment intensification did not lead to

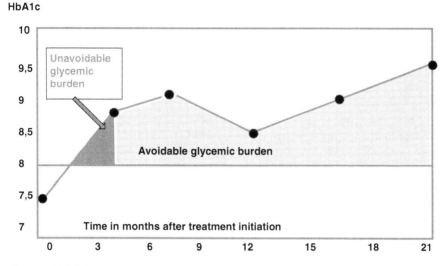

**Fig. 3.1** Risk linked to uncontrolled diabetes: unavoidable and avoidable glycemic burden (From Ref. [17], reproduced with the permission of the American Diabetes Association © 2004)

persistence of elevated blood pressure readings [16]. The authors concluded that certain cases of "clinical inertia" undoubtedly reflected "good clinical judgment".

In diabetes, one can graphically represent the deleterious consequences of persistent poor control by adopting the figure outlined by Brown [17], allowing one to define an "unavoidable glycemic burden" – that linked to poor control appearing between two appointments – and an "avoidable burden", that linked to the fact that HbA1c remained elevated over multiple appointments (Fig. 3.1): this would therefore be a true loss of chance for the patient, if one considers that prolonged poor control is the cause of complications.

Yet Berlowitz also showed in the case of diabetes care, that in a multivariate analysis the greatest predictor of improvement of diabetes control was treatment intensification [6]. The same effect was shown in the recent TRIAD study (Translating Research into Action for Diabetes): of 1,093 uncontrolled diabetic patients, treatment remained unchanged in 573 cases: in the period that followed, HbA1c decreased by 0.36 %; in those whose treatment had been intensified by adding a new oral antidiabetic agent or insulin, it had decreased by 0.73 % or 1.1 %, the improvement of diabetes control being accompanied by weight gain in the case of insulin [18]. Likewise, a study of over 400 diabetic patients showed that lack of treatment intensification, defined as an increase in dose and/or number of medications, even though HbA1c, systolic blood pressure, or LDL-cholesterol remained above 8 %, 140 mmHg, or 1.30 g/l, respectively, was strongly associated with the unfavorable progression of each of these three parameters [19]. More recently, a study using a database of more than 500,000 patients treated in different centers covered by the Kaiser Permanente Northern California Medical Group showed, by comparing the data from different centers, the association between the degree of treatment intensification and improvement of control of diabetes, hypertension and hypercholesterolemia [20]. A study by the same group showed that clinical inertia was more responsible for lack of control of diabetes, hypertension or hyperlipidemia than patient nonadherence: poor adherence was noted in 20–23 % of uncontrolled patients for these three diseases, even though clinical inertia could be at fault in 30, 47, and 36 % of uncontrolled diabetic, hypercholesterolemic and hypertensive patients respectively [21].

Finally, a study clearly showed the importance of prescription (initiation or reinforcement of appropriate treatments) during hospitalization in patients having had a stroke: 6 months later, control of blood pressure and cholesterol was obtained in 41 and 55 % of patients, respectively. Patient adherence to treatment was excellent. A multivariate analysis showed that it was what had been done during the initial hospitalization that was the primary determinant of control of hypertension and hypercholesterolemia [22].

Altogether, this data is consistent with the hypothesis proposed as of 1999 by Cook et al. [23] in the article which used the term clinical inertia for the first time: raising awareness of a team to the concept of clinical inertia as of 1995 was associated both with intensification of treatment and with an improvement over the years of diabetes control. Interestingly enough, this data was obtained within a socially disadvantaged population.

## Analysis of Clinical Inertia in Different Diseases

### Diabetes

The first observation of a delay in implementation or intensification of treatment in diabetes was in fact conducted by this team and published in 1997 with el-Kebbi as first author: in their diabetes clinic in Atlanta, where physicians used a protocol proposing to institute a pharmacological treatment if lifestyle changes were not sufficient to obtain glycemic control (HbA1c remaining above 7 %), this was applied in fact in only 19, 28 and 39 % of follow-up appointments at 2, 4 and 6 months [24]. The same team analyzed in a subsequent study 1,144 appointments. Diabetes control was insufficient in 636 cases. Among these, treatment was not intensified in 146 cases. Yet, physicians were able to correctly identify 88 % of well controlled patients and 94 % of patients whose diabetes control was insufficient. A questionnaire showed that the two reasons most often given for not intensifying treatment were the idea that "control was improving" (34 % of answers), or that patients were adherent to neither their diet nor to the taking of medications (20 % of answers). Interestingly enough, the rate of intensification improved in these patients in the period that followed the carrying out of this survey, which suggests that increasing the awareness of health care providers to the existence of the phenomenon can have a beneficial effect [23, 25].

A study carried out in 2003 in the United States on introduction of metformin treatment in patients insufficiently controlled by hypoglycemic sulfonylureas (in the United States, metformin was accepted by the F.D.A. only relatively recently) revealed that intensification took place only for HbA1c levels above 9 %, and not 8 % as recommended at the time: of 570 patients treated, metformin was introduced on average only 30.2 months after the first observation of HbA1c above 8 % (on average after 4.5 elevated measurements) [26].

A Canadian study, using a database of close to 80,000 diabetic patients, identified 2,652 patients whose diabetes was insufficiently controlled and that could be studied. Comparison of two groups of matched patients, treated by generalists or specialists, showed that treatment intensification took place in fewer than 50 % of appointments. It was a bit more frequent in the case of visits to specialists, but only for starting insulin [27].

However, the study by Ziemer compared the care given in a diabetes clinic (n = 2,157) and a primary care medical clinic (n = 438): treatment intensification in the first case was carried out by a nurse under the supervision of a specialist, in the second by a resident under the supervision of a physician from the center. It was significantly greater in the case of the diabetes clinic, whatever the prescription (diet, oral antidiabetic agents or insulin), and the authors highlighted an association between the degree of intensification and HbA1c [28].

Does practitioner clinical inertia also concern the management of associated risk factors? The situation could in fact be even more serious: in a study of data dating from the end of the 1990s, in 598 type 2 diabetic patients, the treatment had been instituted for 58 % of diabetic patients not yet treated, but only in 34 and 23 %, of hypertension and hypercholesterolemia cases not yet treated, respectively. For patients that were treated, but uncontrolled for each of these factors, intensification took place in 51, 30 and 30 % of appointments, respectively [29].

This was confirmed in a multicentric study of 1,765 patients with type 1 or type 2 diabetes: even though treatment intensification of diabetes took place when faced with uncontrolled HbA1c in 40.6 % of cases, observation of elevated blood pressure or LDL-cholesterol readings led to institution of treatment in only 10.1 and 5.6 % of cases, respectively [30]. The significantly greater clinical inertia in the case of the management of blood pressure and hypercholesterolemia compared to that of diabetes was also highlighted in the study by Wee in Singapore, both in specialists and generalists [31], and in a Dutch study [32]: in the latter, of 3,357 diabetic patients, 161, 875, and 704 patients had their diabetes, their hypertension, or their LDL-cholesterol insufficiently controlled, respectively; the rates of clinical inertia were 35.3, 64.7 and 94.1 %, respectively.

It is possible that this is linked to the number of problems that physicians have to resolve during an appointment whose duration is limited ("competing demands"), which, as we will see, represents one of the generally accepted explanations of clinical inertia: thus, regarding treatment intensification of diabetes itself, a more recent study showed that it was more frequent during a routine visit specifically dedicated to diabetes [33].

## Clinical Inertia in Hospitals

Clinical inertia is not only observed in general practice. Thus, several studies show that diabetes treatment is not intensified faced with elevated glycemic readings in hospitalized patients: for example, in the pilot study by Knecht, treatment was modified in only 34 % of cases [34]; a larger study by the same group, of 2,916 patients even showed that doses of insulin were often *decreased* during hospitalization despite persistent hyperglycemia, perhaps due to the occurrence of an episode of hypoglycemia (what the authors call a "negative therapeutic momentum") [35]. This is perhaps due to the fact that diabetes is often not the primary cause of hospitalization, and that it recedes into the background among treatment priorities [36]. One finds here also the notion of "competing demands", a concept which we will come back to.

A recent study also documented clinical inertia in hospitals, highlighting frequent lack of treatment, prescription of HbA1c testing or organization of remote appointments [37].

## Psychological Insulin Resistance

Introduction of insulin therapy is undoubtedly the most delayed stage of intensification of diabetes management. This is in accordance with what the DAWN (Diabetes Attitudes Wishes and Needs) study showed: physicians often agree with the proposition: "Prefer to delay initiation of insulin therapy until it is absolutely necessary" [38]. Thus, a Canadian study, of 379 type 2 diabetic patients, showed that insulin was introduced for glycated hemoglobin of, on average, 9.5 %, and only 9.2 years after the start of diabetes [39].

In this *"psychological insulin resistance"*, one can typically see a situation in which the physician's and the patient's reasons work together to delay implementation of a treatment which is obviously necessary: the reasons of the one and of the other are at times the same (for example, fear of hypoglycemia and weight gain) [40–42]. One reason given by patients is that they think *"it's the end of the road"* [41], objecting to what they feel is a *"lifelong"* treatment [43]. One understands that psychological insulin resistance often falls under a phenomenon of denial on the part of the patient: in the case of psychological insulin resistance, the clinical inertia of the physician maintains, without knowing it, the patient's denial.

Finally, a study carried out on general practice clearly showed the discordance between the fact that physicians in general agree with the need to obtain good glycemic control to prevent the occurrence of complications from diabetes, and some of their beliefs regarding insulin therapy [44].

## Clinical Inertia and Monitoring of Diabetic Patients

Clinical inertia does not concern only drug prescriptions. Indeed, guidelines specify also the frequency of monitoring tests. These are not optimally prescribed. We'll use as example the recently published study – ENTRED 2007–2010 (*Echantillon national témoin représentatif des personnes diabétiques traitées*), carried out in France and its overseas departments, on the fact that, a diabetic patient has within a year more than 3 HbA1c measures, a measure of each of serum creatinine, proteinuria or microalbuminuria, and blood lipids, and has a cardiology appointment or an electrocardiogram, a dental appointment, and an ophthalmology appointment. Even though the situation has improved a little within the last few years, it is still far from being optimal: for example, though 80 % of patients have an annual measure of serum creatinine, the ophthalmology appointment or the performance of an electrocardiogram are performed in only 40 % of these patients [45].

## Hypertension

We have seen that as of 1998, before the term clinical inertia was even forged, Berlowitz had drawn attention to the fact that hypertensive patients are insufficiently treated [2]. This data was confirmed in several subsequent publications [46–48]. In 2004, Andrade showed that clinical inertia was particularly evident when blood pressure readings were only moderately elevated [49].

Likewise, a recent study of 35,424 patients treated in 428 health centers showed that clinical inertia was significantly greater in cases of so-called "moderate" hypertension [50]. In this study, in a multivariate analysis another determining factor of "therapeutic" inertia (lack of titration of treatment) or even "diagnostic" inertia (lack of initiation of treatment, readings being considered as normal even though they were elevated), was the presence of diabetes, which, again, points in the direction of the concept of "competing demands".

This lack of intensification for "moderately" elevated blood pressure readings was found in the studies by Bolen [51] and by Viera [52]: this data could be explained by the fact that physicians are not sure, for moderately elevated readings, that they actually correspond with uncontrolled hypertension, and we will come back later at length to the role of uncertainty in the birth of clinical inertia. Nevertheless, in the study by Viera [52], lack of treatment intensification was also observed in 46 % of cases where blood pressure readings were at 40 mm above target, therefore in the presence of near certainty.

Lack of compliance with guidelines might not be limited to titration of treatment. Thus, in 2004, a study analyzing 249 patients, treated in 6 health centers and whose hypertension had just been discovered, revealed that hypertension had been diagnosed based on only a single measurement in 85 % of cases, that the electrocardiogram had been performed in only 89 % of cases, that the other routine laboratory tests had been performed in only 50 % of cases, and that after 18 months, 40 % of patients were still under monotherapy [53].

### Description of Barriers to Treatment Intensification in the Case of Hypertension

We have seen that diabetes treatment was more often intensified when the visit was a routine visit [33]. A study by the same team made the same observation for antihypertensive treatment intensification in diabetic patients [51]. In this last study, antihypertensive treatment was less often intensified when glycemia was above 150 mg/dl, which reinforces the role of "competing demands" in the birth of clinical inertia.

Several publications have endeavored to describe the barriers to intensification of care in the field of hypertension [54–57]. When one asks physicians why they did not intensify treatment when faced with elevated blood pressure readings in relation

Analysis of Clinical Inertia in Different Diseases

to guidelines whose existence they are aware of, the reasons most often mentioned are uncertainty on the reality of elevated blood pressure readings, the fact that the readings are improving and that it is too soon to make a decision, patient nonadherence, the fact that the management of hypertension is difficult, especially in diabetic patients, and lack of time during appointments that are too short, where hypertension was not a priority [57].

## Hyperlipidemia

Lack of treatment of hypercholesterolemia, or lack of titration of the prescription of the dose of statin until the LDL-cholesterol target set based on the number of risk factors is reached, was an integral part of Phillips' initial observations which had led him to forge the term clinical inertia [58], and of the study by Rodondi [1], which we have previously cited. Subsequently, several publications have shown the insufficiency of prescription of statin despite publication of precise Guidelines such as those by the National Cholesterol Education Program (NCEP) [59, 60] in 2007; in a study of 2,103 appointments of patients not having reached the target and not on a maximum dose of statin, treatment was intensified in only 16 % of cases [61].

In this study, a multivariate analysis showed that intensification was more frequent in cases of particularly elevated LDL-cholesterol readings and in adherent patients, less frequent in elderly or diabetic patients, as we have already observed for treatment of diabetes and hypertension [61]. This effect of the level of LDL-cholesterol was also observed in a small cohort of hypercholesterolemic patients with HIV, where clinical inertia was observed in 44 % of cases, with a greater rate of inertia in women [62]. The recent study by Lazaro, which we have previously cited [7], in which a 43 % rate of clinical inertia was observed, also showed the high rate of clinical inertia in treatment of hypercholesterolemic women, an effect also observed in the study by Abuful [63].

We will come back in the following chapter to the reasons for this difference in management linked to sex, clearly analyzed in the review by Kim et al. [64].

## Cardiovascular Risk Prevention

More generally, a recent study carried out in Australia on cardiovascular risk prevention in coronary heart disease patients made it possible to illustrate the often insufficient treatment in terms of prescription of antihypertensive and hypolipidemic medication and antiplatelet agents: of 1,548 patients who had cardiovascular disease, only 50 % received a combination associating these three medications; treatment intensification depended on the assessment of risk, but remained at times insufficient even in cases of high risk, established with the Framingham Risk Score [65].

The study by Mosca also showed that the level of prescription depended, as it should, on assessment of risk. Nevertheless, practitioners often underestimated the vascular risk of patients, especially in women [66].

## Other Conditions Where One Can Highlight the Clinical Inertia Phenomenon

### Heart Failure

Several studies have endeavored to describe compliance of health care providers with guidelines in this field. Thus, in the EuroHeart Failure Survey Program, published in 2003, of close to 50,000 patients, over 90 % of them had actually had at the time of their admission to hospital an electrocardiogram, a chest x-ray, a hemoglobin measure and an electrolyte test, as recommended by the European Society of Cardiology, but only 66 % of patients had had an echocardiogram [67]. Regarding treatment, only 17 % of patients received the recommended triple association of diuretics, angiotensin-converting-enzyme inhibitors (ACE inhibitors) and beta-blockers [68]. This data confirms the results of the IMPROVEMENT of Heart Failure Program study, published the previous year, of 11,062 patients treated by general practitioners: most of the practitioners knew the benefits of ACE inhibitors and beta-blockers; yet, only 60 % of patients received ACE inhibitors, 34 % received beta-blockers, and 20 % received both medications, doses being below the recommended doses [69].

Two more recent studies have shown that guideline compliance represents a determining factor in the prognosis of these patients: for example, the MAHLER (Medical Management of Chronic Heart Failure in Europe and its Related Costs) study constructed a class adherence indicator (GAI3) to three drug classes: ACE inhibitors, diuretics and beta-blockers. An association with the rate of hospitalization was clearly highlighted. Noncompliance with guidelines was in a multivariate analysis an independent factor explaining the risk of hospitalization, just like the degree of heart failure, a history of hospitalization, an ischemic etiology of heart failure, and the presence of diabetes and hypertension [70]. More recently, an Israeli study showed that following guidelines for patients hospitalized for an episode of heart failure in an internal medicine unit, leading especially to an increase in the performance of ultrasounds and prescription of ACE inhibitors and beta-blockers, was associated with a decrease in mortality of patients at 3 months [71].

### Management of Valvular Heart Disease

Two studies have shown that the management of valvular heart disease was not always carried out in accordance with guidelines: thus, regarding aortic valve disease, the Euro Heart Survey on Valvular Heart Disease, published in 2007, assessed medical practices in 136 patients with severe, isolated, and asymptomatic aortic valve disease. The decision to operate was compared with guidelines by the American College of Cardiology/American Heart Association. It was in accordance with guidelines in 68 % of cases of aortic stenosis and in 83 % of cases of aortic insufficiency: an excessive indication was noted in 21 % of cases of stenosis and in 9 % of cases of aortic insufficiency, and an insufficient indication was noted in 11 % of cases of stenosis and in 8 % of cases of aortic insufficiency [72]. Another study showed that older patient age and a poor systolic ejection fraction represented two significant factors explaining the refusal to operate patients with severe aortic stenosis, even though data from the literature suggests that, certainly operative risk increases with age, but that age is not predictive of long-term survival, which led clinical practice guidelines to propose that age in and of itself is not a contraindication for the intervention [73].

Likewise, in the case of mitral regurgitation, the Euro Heart Survey on Valvular Heart Disease revealed that in 101 asymptomatic patients with non-ischemic severe mitral regurgitation, the decision to operate was in accordance with guidelines in 62 % of cases, with an operative indication considered "excessive" in 9 patients, and "insufficient" in 29 patients in relation to guidelines [74].

## Complete Arrhythmia Due to Atrial Fibrillation

Despite accumulation of evidence in favor of the beneficial effect of treatment of complete arrhythmia due to atrial fibrillation with anticoagulants in patients at high risk of stroke, this type of treatment remains insufficiently used. For example, the Euro Heart Survey of AF Patients [75] showed that only 67 % of patients in principle eligible were treated with anticoagulants. Nevertheless, guidelines also ask to consider risk level; yet this study also showed that patients that could be considered as *at low risk* of stroke received anticoagulant treatment, contrary to guidelines.

These deviations from guidelines have consequences: in patients considered as being at high risk, 28 % of patients were insufficiently treated, and 11 % were overtreated according to guidelines; the insufficiency of treatment was associated with an increased risk of occurrence of a thromboembolic event (Relative Risk 1.97, 95 % Confidence Interval: 1.29–3.01); over treatment was associated non significantly with an increased risk of bleeding (RR 1.52, 95 % CI: 0.76–3.02) [76].

Two studies show that physicians have the tendency to under treat with anticoagulants patients with AF when they have experienced a case of bleeding induced by the treatment, while their practice is not modified in favor of treatment by the memory of a case of embolic event in an untreated patient [77, 78]. We will comment later on this preference for errors of omission, over errors of commission.

## Asthma

As of 2000, a literature review described the "gap" between guidelines and clinical practice in the field of asthma [79]. Thus, a study analyzed precisely, for each of the guidelines which had been published in 1997 by the National Heart, Lung, and Blood Institute, the nature of barriers identified by pediatricians to their implementation: for example, regarding the use of inhaled corticosteroids, it highlighted lack of familiarity with this type of treatment, disagreement with the guideline, lack of mastery of the treatment, and the idea that it would not be used by the child or her parents [80]. A study carried out in 2003–2004 in Scotland, a country where asthma is particularly frequent, again revealed that less than a quarter of patients had received patient education describing "a therapeutic action plan", even though this is an integral part of the guidelines. Regarding specifically this guideline, 98.4 % of physicians questioned claimed to know it, 79.7 % agreed with the idea that its implementation would bring about better management of patients, but 46 % thought

24          3 The Evidence: The Gap Between Guidelines and Clinical Reality

that its implementation required a reorganization of patient care. In fact, an audit showed that it was followed for only 22.8 % of patients [81].

On this specific point, implementation of guidelines in the form of a leaflet at the time of admission to hospital for an asthma attack can be effective: a recent Australian study compared the management of children with asthma before and after this measure: afterwards, an action plan was given twice as often (23 vs. 11 % of cases, p = 0.0003) [82].

Although asthma had been used at first as an example of a disease in which the issue of the discordance between guidelines and clinical practice arises [80, 83, 84], it is relatively difficult to find in the literature an estimation of the amplitude of clinical inertia in this field. Perhaps this is due to the fact that the concept of unequivocal guidelines and their applicability can be criticized faced with the heterogeneity of asthma [85].

## Osteoporosis

A recent literature review shows that management of osteoporosis is also very often insufficient [86]. Thus, a Belgian study published in 2008 showed that, among 23,146 patients having had a hip fracture, only 6 % of them had received treatment, mainly with bisphosphonate [87]; likewise, a Danish study of 152,777 fractures showed that after a hip fracture, in 2004, treatment with bisphosphonate was instituted in only 9.2 % of women and 4.1 % of men, values being 39.6 % and 16.5 % after a vertebral compression fracture [88]. Lack of treatment was found more frequently in elderly patients [89].

It has also been shown that screening for osteoporosis in elderly men is insufficient [90] and that physicians often do not implement preventive treatment of osteoporosis during long term corticotherapy [91, 92]. The barriers most often put forth by physicians were lack of awareness of guidelines, the presence of other priorities, the limited time of appointments, barriers relating to the patient – the fact that it is a silent disease, poor patient adherence, the presence of comorbidities -, and finally, barriers relating to the health care system – for example the difficulty of obtaining a bone mineral density test [91].

A German study published in 2007, of 2,194 general practitioners, showed that among the 892 practitioners who answered the questionnaire, 82.7 % thought themselves competent in the management of osteoporosis, 51.7 % were well aware of the existence of guidelines, and 43 % used them without problem. Often, physicians stated that budgetary restrictions represented a significant obstacle to the prescription of recommended treatments [93].

*

* *

We could continue to give countless examples: the clinical inertia phenomenon was also highlighted in the management of depression [94], screening for colon cancer [95], prescription of nonsteroidal anti-inflammatory drugs [96] etc. The *Revue Médicale de Liège* devoted in 2010 a special issue to clinical inertia, and one will find here an analysis of the literature in fields as diverse as, for example, quitting smoking [97], contraception [98], and obstetrics [99]. Intelligently, most articles associate the issue of physician clinical inertia with that of patient nonadherence [100]. More recently, the French journal *Médecine des Maladies Métaboliques* devoted a special issue to the subject of clinical inertia and its significance in contemporary medicine [101].

Thus, the preceding data leads one to acknowledge what is in fact a truism: each time that a guideline is put forward in a particular field, it may occur that it is not followed. As we have insisted from the onset, this may be an *appropriate inaction* on the part of the physician. Nevertheless, we have cited examples where this occurs in more than half of cases: unless one challenges the validity, even the very principle of guidelines, and, consequently, the new medical state of mind, to not use the term "new paradigm", that Evidence-Based Medicine represents, one must admit that some of these inactions fall under inertia, such as we have defined it.

In summary, it seems that what one could call true clinical inertia is a reality in medicine and that its frequency and consequences make it a major public health problem. If one hopes to be able to resolve it, it is necessary to understand on an individual level the birth of a phenomenon which appears so ubiquitous: one must therefore pass from epidemiological descriptions to mechanisms liable to explain it at the level of physician behavior.

## References

1. Rodondi N, Peng T, Karter AJ, Bauer DC, Vittinghoff E, Tang S, Pettitt D, Kerr EA, Selby JV. Therapy modifications in response to poorly controlled hypertension, dyslipidemia, and diabetes mellitus. Ann Intern Med. 2006;144:475–84.
2. Berlowitz DR, Ash AS, Hickey E, Friedman RRH, Glickman M, Kader B, Moskowitz MA. Inadequate management of blood pressure in a hypertensive population. N Engl J Med. 1998;339:1957–63.
3. Okonofua EC, Simpson KN, Jesri A, Durkalski VL, Egan BM. Therapeutic inertia is an impediment to achieving the healthy people 2010 blood pressure control goals. Hypertension. 2006;47:345–51.
4. Balkau B, Bouée S, Avignon A, Vergès B, Chartier I, Amelineau E, Halimi S. Type 2 diabetes treatment intensification in general practice in France in 2008–2009: The DIAttitude study. Diabetes Metab. 2012;38 Suppl 3:S29–35.
5. Simon D. Therapeutic inertia in type 2 diabetes: insights from the PANORAMA study in France. Diabetes Metab. 2012;38 Suppl 3:S47–52.
6. Berlowitz DR, Ash AS, Glickman M, Friedman RH, Pogach LM, Nelson AL, Wong AT. Developing a quality measure for clinical inertia in diabetes care. Health Res Educ Trust. 2005;40:1836–51.
7. Lazaro P, Murga N, Aguilar D, Hernandez-Presa MA. Therapeutic Inertia in the outpatient management of dyslipidemia in patients with ischemic heart disease. The inertia study. Rev Esp Cardiol. 2010;63:1428–37.
8. Kerr EA, Smith DM, Hogan MM, Hofer TP, Krein SR, Bermann M, Hayward RA. Building a better quality measure. Are some patients with "poor quality" actually getting good care ? Med Care. 2003;41:1173–82.
9. Gil-Guillén V, Orozco-Beltrán D, Carratalá-Munuera C, Márquez-Contreras E, Durazo-Arvizu R, Cooper R, Pertusa-Martínez S, Pita-Fernandez S, González-Segura D, Martin-de-Pablo JL, Pallarés V, Fernández A, Redón J. Clinical inertia in poorly controlled elderly hypertensive patients: a cross-sectional study in spanish physicians to ascertain reasons for not intensifying treatment. Am J Cardiovasc Drugs. 2013;13:213–9.

10. Nelson SAE, Dresser GK, Vandervoort MK, Wong CJ, Feagan BG, Mahon JL, Feldman RD. Barriers to blood pressure control: a STITCH substudy. J Clin Hypertens (Greenwich). 2011;13:73–80.
11. Green BB, Cook AJ, Ralston JD, et al. Effectiveness of home blood pressure monitoring, web communication, and pharmacist care on hypertension control: a randomized controlled trial. JAMA. 2008;299:2857–67.
12. Simpson SH, Majumdar SR, Tsuyuki RT, et al. Effect of adding pharmacists to primary care teams on blood pressure control in patients with type 2 diabetes: a randomized controlled trial. Diabetes Care. 2011;34:20–6.
13. Rinfret S, Lussier MT, Peirce A, et al. The impact of a multidisciplinary information tech-nologysupported program on blood pressure control in primary care. Circ Cardiovasc Qual Outcomes. 2009;2:170–7.
14. Luders S, Schrader J, Schmieder RE, Smolka W, Wegscheider K, Bestehorn K. Improvement o hypertension management by structured physician education and feedback system: cluster randomized trial. Eur J Cardiovasc Prev Rehabil. 2010;17:271–9.
15. Huebschmann AG, Mizrahi T, Soenksen A, Beaty BL, Denberg TD. Reducing clinical inertia in hypertension treatment: a pragmatic randomized controlled trial. J Clin Hypertens (Greenwich). 2012;14:322–9.
16. Crowley MJ, Smith VA, Olsen MK, Danus S, Oddone EZ, Bosworth HB, Powers BJ. Treatment intensification in a hypertension telemangement trial. Clinical inertia or good clinical judgment ? Hypertension. 2011;58:552–8.
17. Brown JB, Nichols GA, Perry A. The burden of treatment failure in type 2 diabetes. Diabetes Care. 2004;27:1535–40.
18. McEwen LN, Johnson SL, Halter JB, Karter AJ, Mangione CM, Subramanian U, Waitzfelder B, Crosson JC, Herman WH. Predictors and impact of intensification of antihyperglycemic therapy in type 2 diabetes. Translating Research into Action for Diabetes (TRIAD). Diabetes Care. 2009;32:971–6.
19. Samuels TA, Bolen S, Yeh HC, Abuid M, Marinopoulos SS, Weiner JP, McGuire M, Brancati FL. Missed opportunities in diabetes management: a longitudinal assessment of factors asso-ciated with sub-optimal quality. J Gen Intern Med. 2008;23:1770–7.
20. Selby JV, Uratzu CS, Fireman B, Schmittdiel JA, Peng T, Rodondi N, Karter A, Kerr EA. Treatment intensification and risk factor control: Toward more clinically relevant quality measures. Med Care. 2009;47:395–402.
21. Schmittdiel JA, Uratsu CS, Karter AJ, Heisler M, Subramanian U, Mangione CM, Selby JV. Why don't diabetes patients achieve recommended risk factor targets? Poor adherence versus lack of treatment intensification. J Gen Intern Med. 2008;23:588–94.
22. Touzé E, Coste J, Voicu M, Kansao J, Masmoudi R, Doumenc B, Durieux P, Mas JL. Importance of in-hospital initiation of therapies and therapeutic inertia in secondary stroke prevention. Implementation of Prevention After a Cerebrovascular evenT (IMPACT) study. Stroke. 2008;39:1834–43.
23. Cook CB, Ziemer DC, El-Kebbi IM, Gallina DL, Dunbar VG, Ernst KL, Phillips LS. Diabetes in urban African-Americans. XVI. Overcoming clinical inertia improves glycemic control in patients with type 2 diabetes. Diabetes Care. 1999;22:1494–500.
24. El-Kebbi IM, Ziemer DC, Musey VC, Gallina DL, Bernard AM, Phillips LS. Diabetes in urban African-Americans. IX Provider adherence to management protocols. Diabetes Care. 1997;20:698–703.
25. El-Kebbi IM, Ziemer DC, Gallina DL, Dunbar V, Phillips LS. Diabetes in urban African-Americans. XV Identification of barriers to provider adherence to management protocols. Diabetes Care. 1999;22:1617–20.
26. Brown JB, Nichols GA. Slow response to loss of glycemic control in type 2 diabetes mellitus. Am J Manag Care. 2003;9:213–7.
27. Shah BJ, Hux JE, Laupacis A, Zinman B, van Walraven C. Clinical inertia in response to inadequate glycemic control. Do specialists differ from primary care physicians? Diabetes Care. 2005;28:600–6.

# References

27

28. Ziemer DC, Miller CD, Rhee MK, Doyle JP, Watkins Jr C, Cook CB, Gallina DL, El-Kebbi IM, Barnes CS, Dunbar VG, Branch Jr WT, Phillips LS. Clinical inertia contributes to poor diabetes control in a primary care setting. Diabetes Educ. 2005;31:564–71.
29. Grant RW, Caglero E, Dubey AK, Gildesgame C, Chueh HC, Barry MJ, Singer DE, Nathan DM, Meigs JB. Clinical inertia in the management of type 2 diabetes metabolic risk factors. Diabet Med. 2004;21:150–5.
30. Grant RW, Buse JB, Meigs JB. Quality of diabetes care in U.S. academic medical centers. Diabetes Care. 2005;28:337–442.
31. Wee SL, Tan CG, Ng HS, Su C, Tai VU, Flores JVPG, Kho DHC. Diabetes outcome in specialist and general practitioner settings in Singapore: challenges of right-siting. Ann Acad Med Singapore. 2008;37:929–35.
32. Van Bruggen R, Gorter K, Stolk R, Klungel O, Rutten G. Clinical inertia in general practice: widespread and related to the outcome of diabetes care. Fam Pract. 2009;26:428–36.
33. Bolen SD, Bricker E, Samuels TA, Yeh HC, Marinopoulos SS, McGuire M, Abuid M, Brancati FL. Factors associated with intensification of oral diabetes medications in primary care provider-patient dyads: a cohort study. Diabetes Care. 2009;32:25–31.
34. Knecht LA, Gauthier SM, Castro JC, Schmidt RE, Whitaker MD, Zimmerman RS, Mishark KJ, Cook CB. Diabetes care in the hospital: is there clinical inertia? J Hosp Med. 2006;1:151–60.
35. Cook CB, Castro JC, Schmidt RE, Whitaker MD, Roust LR, Argueta R, Hull BP, Zimmerman RS. Diabetes care in hospitalized non critically ill patients: more evidence for clinical inertia and negative therapeutic momentum. J Hosp Med. 2007;2:203–11.
36. Cook CB, Zimmerman RS, Gauthier SM, Castro JC, Jameson KA, Littman SD, Magallanez JM. Understanding and improving management of inpatient diabetes mellitus: the Mayo Clinic Arizona experience. J Diabetes Sci Technol. 2008;2:925–31.
37. Griffith ML, Boord JB, Eden SK, Matheny ME. Clinical inertia of discharge planning among patients with poorly controlled diabetes mellitus. J Clin Endocrinol Metab. 2012;97:2019–26.
38. Peyrot M, Rubin RR, Lauritzen T, Skovlund SE, Snoek FJ, Matthews DR, Landgraf R, Kleinebreil L, International DAWN Advisory Panel. Resistance to insulin therapy among patients and providers: results of the cross-national Diabetes Attitudes, Wishes, and Needs (DAWN) study. Diabetes Care. 2005;28:2673–9.
39. Harris SB, Kapor J, Lank CN, Willan AR, Houston T. Clinical inertia in patients with T2DM requiring insulin in family practice. Can Fam Physician. 2010;56:e418–24.
40. Leslie CA, Satin-Rapaport W, Matheson D, Stone R, Enfield G. Psychological insulin resistance: a missed diagnosis. Diab Spectr. 1994;7:52–7.
41. Phillips P. Type 2 diabetes – failure, blame and guilt in the adoption of insulin therapy. Rev Diab Stud. 2005;2:35–9.
42. Peyrot M, Rubin RR, Khunti K. Addressing barriers to initiation of insulin in patients with type 2 diabetes. Prim Care Diabetes. 2010;4 Suppl 1:11–8.
43. Woudenberg YJ, Lucas C, Latour C, Scholte O, Reimer WJ. Acceptance of insulin therapy: a long shot? Psychological insulin resistance in primary care. Diabet Med. 2012;29:796–802.
44. Hayes RP, Fitzgerald JT, Jacober SJ. Primary care physician beliefs about insulin initiation in patients with type 2 diabetes. Int J Clin Pract. 2008;62:860–8.
45. Ndong JR, Romon I, Druet C, Prévot L, Hubert-Brierre R, Pascolini E, Thomaset JP, Cheungkin R, Bravo A, Chantry M, Deligne J, Paumier A, Weill A, Fagot-Campana A. Caractéristiques, risque vasculaire, complications et qualité des soins des personnes diabétiques dans les départements d'outre-mer et comparaison à la métropole: Entred 2007–2010, France. BEH. 2010;42–43:432–6.
46. Alexander M, Tekawa I, Hunkeler E, Fireman B, Rowell R, Selby JV, Massie BM, Cooper W. Evaluating hypertension control in a managed care setting. Arch Intern Med. 1999;159:2673–7.
47. Knight EL, Bohn RL, Wang PS, Glynn RJ, Mogun H, Avorn J. Predictors of uncontrolled hypertension in ambulatory patients. Hypertension. 2001;38:809–14.

48. Oliveria SA, Lapuerta P, McCarthy BD, L'Italien GJ, Berlowitz DR, Ash SM. Physician-related barriers to the effective management of uncontrolled hypertension. Arch Intern Med. 2002;162:413–20.

49. Andrade SE, Gurwitz JH, Field TS, Kelleher M, Majumdar SR, Reed G, Black R. Hypertension management: the care gap between clinical guidelines and clinical practice. Am J Manag Care. 2004;10:481–6.

50. Gil-Guillén V, Orozco-Beltran D, Pérez RP, Alfonso JL, Redon J, Pertusa-Martinez S, Navarro J, Cea-Calvo L, Quirce-Andres F, Merino-Sanchez J, Carratala C, Martin-Moreno JM. Clinical inertia in diagnosis and treatment of hypertension in primary care: quantification and association factors. Blood Press. 2010;19:3–10.

51. Bolen SD, Samuels TA, Yeh HC, Marnopoulos SS, McGuire M, Abuid M, Brancati FL. Failure to intensify antihypertensive treatmenet by primary care providers: a cohort study in adults with diabetes mellitus and hypertension. J Gen Intern Med. 2008;23:543–50.

52. Viera AJ, Schmid D, Bostrom S, Yow A, Lawrence W, DuBard CA. Level of blood pressure above goal and clinical inertia in a medicaid population. J Am Soc Hypertens. 2010;4:244–54.

53. Spranger CB, Ries A, Berge CA, Radford NB, Victor RG. Identifying gaps between guidelines and clinical practice in the evaluation and treatment of patients with hypertension. Am J Med. 2004;117:14–8.

54. Lin ND, Martins SB, Chan AS, Coleman RW, Bosworth HB, Oddone EZ, Shankar RD, Musen MA, Hoffman BB, Goldstein MK. Identifying barriers to hypertension guideline adherence using clinician feedback at the point of care. AMIA 2006 symposium proceedings. AMIA Symposium, American Medical Informatics Association. 2006. p. 494–8.

55. Bramlage P, Thoenes M, Kirch W, Lenfant C. Clinical practice and recent recommendations in hypertension management –reporting a gap in a global survey of 1259 primary care physicians in 17 countries. Curr Med Res Opin. 2007;23:783–91.

56. Holland N, Segraves D, Nnadi VO, Belletti DA, Wogen J, Arcona S. Identifying barriers to hypertension care: implications for quality improvement initiatives. Dis Manag. 2008;11:71–7.

57. Ferrari P. Reasons for therapeutic inertia when managing hypertension in clinical practice in non-western countries. J Hum Hypertens. 2009;23:151–9.

58. Phillips LS, Branch WT, Cook CB, Doyle JP, El-Kebbi IM, Gallina DL, Miller CD, Ziemer DC, Barnes CS. Clinical inertia. Ann Intern Med. 2001;135:825–34.

59. McBride P, Schrott HG, Plane MB, Underbakke G, Brown RL. Primary care adherence to national cholesterol education program guidelines for patients with coronary heart disease. Arch Intern Med. 1998;158:1238–44.

60. Pearson T, Laurora I, Chu H, Kafonek S. The lipid treatment assessment project (L-TAP): a multicenter survey to evaluate the percentages of dyslipidemic patients receiving lipid-lowering therapy and achieving low-density lipoprotein cholesterol goals. Arch Intern Med. 2000;160:459–67.

61. Goldberg KC, Melnyk SD, Simel DL. Overcoming inertia: improvement in achieving target low-density lipoprotein cholesterol. Am J Manag Care. 2007;13:530–4.

62. Willig JH, Jacson DA, Westfall AO, Allison J, Chang PW, Raper J, Saag MS, Mugavero MJ. Clinical inertia in the management of low-density lipoprotein abnormalities in an HIV clinic. Clin Infect Dis. 2008;46:1315–8.

63. Abuful A, Gidron Y, Henkin Y. Physicians' attitudes toward preventive therapy for coronary artery disease: is there a gender bias? Clin Cardiol. 2005;28:389–93.

64. Kim C, Hofer T, Kerr EA. Review of evidence and explanations for suboptimal screening and treatment of dyslipidemia in women. A conceptual model. J Gen Intern Med. 2003;18:854–63.

65. Heeley EL, Peiris DP, Patel AA, Cass A, Weekes A, Morgan C, Anderson CS, Chalmers JP. Cardiovascular risk perception and evidence-practice gaps in Australian general practice (the AusHEART study). Med J Aust. 2010;192:254–9.

66. Mosca L, Linfante AH, Benjamin EJ, Berra K, Hayes SN, Walsh BW, Fabunmi RP, Kwan J, Mills T, Simpson SL. National study of physician awareness and adherence to cardiovascular disease prevention guidelines. Circulation. 2005;111:499–510.

67. Cleland JGF, Swedberg K, Follath F, Komadja M, Cohen-Solal A, Aguilar JC, Dietz R, Gavazzi A, Hobbs R, Korewicki J, Madeira HC, Moiseyev VS, Predam I, van Gilst WH, Widimsk J, Freemantle N, Eastaugh J, Mason J. The EuroHeart Failure survey programme—a survey on the quality of care among patients with heart failure in Europe part 1: patient characteristics and diagnosis. Eur Heart J. 2003;24:442–63.
68. Komajda M, Follath F, Swedberg K, Cleland J, Aguilar JC, Cohen-Solal A, Dietz R, Gavazzi A, Van Gilst WH, Hobbs R, Korewicki J, Madeira HC, Moiseyev VS, Preda I, Widimsky J, Freemantle N, Eastaugh J, Mason J. The EuroHeart failure survey programme—a survey on the quality of care among patients with heart failure in Europe. Part 2: treatment. Eur Heart J. 2003;24:464–74.
69. Cleland JGF, Cohen-Solal A, Aguilar JC, Dietz R, Eastaugh J, Follath F, Freemantle N, Gavazzi A, van Gilst WH. Management of heart failure in primary care (the IMPROVEMENT of heart failure programme): an international survey. Lancet. 2002;360:1631–9.
70. Komajda M, Lapuerta P, Hermans N, Gonzalez-Juanatey JR, van Veldhuisen DJ, Erdmann E, Tavazzi L, Poole-Wilson P, Le Pen C. Adherence to guidelines is a predictor of outcome in chronic heart failure: the MAHLER survey. Eur Heart J. 2005;26:1653–9.
71. Braun E, Landsman K, Zuckerman R, Berger G, Meilik A, Azzam ZS. Adherence to guidelines improves the clinical outcome of patients with acutely decompensated heart failure. IMAJ. 2009;11:348–53.
72. Iung B, Messika-Zeitoun D, Cachier A, Delahaye F, Baron G, Tornos P, Gohlke-Bärwolf C, Boersma E, Ravaud P, Vahanian A. Actual management of patients with asymptomatic aortic valve disease: how practice fits with guidelines. Am Heart J. 2007;153:696–703.
73. Iung B, Cachier A, Baron G, Messika-Zeitoun D, Delahaye F, Tornos P, Gohlke-Bärwolf C, Boersma E, Ravaud P, Vahanian A. Decision-making in elderly patients with severe aortic stenosis: why are so many denied surgery? Eur Heart J. 2005;26:2714–20.
74. Detaint D, Iung B, Lepage L, Messika-Zeitoun D, Baron G, Tornos P, Gohlke-Bärwolf C, Vahanian A. Management of asymptomatic patients with severe non-ischaemic mitral regurgitation. Are practices consistent with guidelines? Eur J Cardiothorac Surg. 2008;34:937–42.
75. Nieuwlaat R, Capucci A, Lip GY, Olsson SB, Prins MH, Nieman FH, Lopez-Sendon J, Vardas PE, Aliot E, Santini M, Crijns HJ. Antithrombotic treatment in real-life atrial fibrillation patients: a report from the Euro Heart Survey on Atrial Fibrillation. Eur Heart J. 2006;27:3018–26.
76. Nieuwlaat R, Olsson SB, Lip GY, Camm AJ, Breithardt G, Capucci A, Meeder JG, Prins MH, Lévy S, Crijns HJ. Guideline-adherent antithrombotic treatment is associated with improved outcomes compared with undertreatment in high-risk patients with atrial fibrillation. The Euro Heart Survey on Atrial Fibrillation. Am Heart J. 2007;153:1006–12.
77. Gattellari M, Worthington J, Zwar N, Middleton S. Barriers to the use of anticoagulation for nonvalvular atrial fibrillation: a representative survey of Australian family physicians. Stroke. 2008;39:227–30.
78. Choudhry NK, Anderson GM, Laupacis A, Ross-Degnan D, Normand SLT, Soumerai SB. Impact of adverse events on prescribing warfarin in patients with atrial fibrillation: matched pair analysis. BMJ. doi:10.1136/bmj.38698.709572.55.
79. Crim C. Clinical practice guidelines vs actual clinical practice. The asthma paradigm. Chest. 2000;118:62S–4.
80. Cabana MD, Ebel BE, Cooper-Patrick L, Powe NR, Rubin HR, Rand CS. Barriers pediatricians face when using asthma guidelines. Arch Pediatr Adolesc Med. 2000;154:683–93.
81. Wiener-Ogielvie S, Pinnock H, Huby G, Sheikh A, Partridge MR, Gillies J. Do practices comply with key recommendations of the British Asthma Guideline? If not, why not ? Prim Care Respir J. 2007;116:369–77.
82. Gildenhuys J, Lee M, Isbister GK. Does implementation of a paediatric asthma clinical practice guideline worksheet change clinical practice? Int J Emerg Med. 2009;2:33–9.
83. Cabana MD, Flores G. The role of clinical practice guidelines in enhancing quality and reducing racial/ethnic disparities in paediatrics. Paediatr Respir Rev. 2002;3:52–8.

84. Byrnes P, McGoldrick C, Crawford M. Asthma cycle of care attendance. Overcoming therapeutic inertia using an asthma clinic. Aust Fam Physician. 2010;39:318–20.
85. Price D, Thomas M. Breaking new ground: challenging existing asthma guidelines. BMC Pulm Med. 2006;6 Suppl 1:S6. doi:10.1186/1471-2466-6-S1-S6.
86. Rabenda V, Reginster JY. Prévention et traitement de l'ostéoporose: éviter l'inertie clinique et motiver l'adhésion au traitement. Rev Med Liege. 2010;65:358–65.
87. Rabenda V, Vanoverloop J, Fanbri V, Mertens R, Sumkay F, Vannecke C, Deswaef A, Verpooten GA, Reginster JY. Low incidence of anti-osteoporosis treatment after hip fracture. J Bone Joint Surg Am. 2008;90:2142–8.
88. Roerholt C, Eiken P, Abrahamsen B. Initiation of anti-osteoporotic therapy in patients with recent fractures: a nationwide analysis of prescription rates and persistence. Osteoporos Int. 2009;20:299–307.
89. Feldstein AC, Nichols GA, Elmer PJ, Smith DH, Aickin M, Herson M. Older women with fractures: patients falling through the cracks of guideline-recommended osteoporosis screening and treatment. J Bone Joint Surg Am. 2003;85-A:2294–302.
90. Cheng N, Green ME. Osteoporosis screening for men. Are family physicians following the guidelines? Can Fam Physician. 2008;54:1140–1.e1–5.
91. Guzman-Clark JR, Fang MA, Sehl ME, Traylor L, Hahn TJ. Barriers in the management of glucocorticoid-induced osteoporosis. Arthritis Rheum. 2007;57:140–6.
92. Feldstein AC, Elmer PJ, Nichols GA, Herson M. Practice patterns in patients at risk for glucocorticoid-induced osteoporosis. Osteoporos Int. 2005;16:2168–74.
93. Chenot R, Scheidt-Nave C, Gabler S, Kochen MM, Himmel W. German primary care doctors' awareness of osteoporosis and knowledge of national guidelines. Exp Clin Endocrinol Diabetes. 2007;115:584–9.
94. Henke RM, Zaslavsky AM, McGuire TG, Ayanian JZ, Rubenstein LV. Clinical inertia in depression treatment. Med Care. 2009;47:959–67.
95. Guerra CE, Schwartz JS, Armstrong K, Brown JS, Halbert CH, Shea JA. Barriers of and facilitators to physician recommendation of colorectal cancer screening. J Gen Intern Med. 2007;22:1681–8.
96. Cavazos JM, Naik AD, Woofter A, Abraham S. Barriers to physician adherence to nonsteroidal anti-inflammatory drug guidelines: a qualitative study. Aliment Pharmacol Ther. 2008;28:789–98.
97. Deflandre E, Degey S, Clerdain AM, Jaucot J, Joris J, Brichant JF. Sevrage tabagique en préopératoire: une période propice pour lutter contre l'inertie et le défaut d'observance. Rev Med Liege. 2010;65:332–7.
98. Pintiaux A, Bouuaert C, Habay N, Beliard A, Foidart JM, Nisolle M. L'inertie thérapeutique en contraception. Rev Med Liege. 2010;65:2391–4.
99. Masson V, Petit P, Foidart JM. Défaut d'observance et inertie thérapeutique en obstétrique. Rev Med Liege. 2010;65:395–8.
100. Scheen AJ, Giet D. Editorial. Cibler l'inertie et le défaut d'observance thérapeutiques: nouveau défi pour améliorer les performances de la pratique médicale. Rev Med Liege. 2010;65:229–31.
101. Reach G. Éditorial, Inertie clinique: ce que révèle le concept. Médecine Mal Métaboliques. 2011;5 Suppl 2:S43–5.

# Determinants and Explanatory Models of Clinical Inertia

**4**

## Abstract

In their initial publication, Phillips et al. proposed three main explanations of clinical inertia: denial, the use of soft reasons (the situation is improving, or, the patient is nonadherent anyway), and lack of physician training in the concept of treatment titration. Since then, other factors have been highlighted: uncertainty regarding the actual state of the patient (in particular blood pressure), and competing demands which draw the physician's attention to acute issues, to the detriment of prevention measures. In this chapter we also analyze other reasons, such as the characteristics of the physicians, the fact that the patient belongs to an ethnic minority or is disadvantaged, and finally the relationship between physician clinical inertia and patient nonadherence. In the second part of this chapter, we discuss several theoretical models of clinical inertia, including the Knowledge–Attitude-Behavior-Result model described by Cabana, The Awareness-Agreement-Adoption-Adherence model, the Physician Guideline Compliance model, and the application to the clinical inertia issue of the Regulatory Focus Theory by Higgins, proposed by Veazie.

Observation of a gap between the ideal world of clinical practice guidelines and clinical practice reality quickly led to reflection upon the reasons which can bring about clinical inertia, or, more generally, physician noncompliance regarding guidelines which were nevertheless widely disseminated.

In the case of patient nonadherence regarding medical prescriptions, one can describe determinants of the phenomenon and even propose to construct explanatory models of nonadherent behavior (for example the Health Belief Model, the Transtheoretical Model of Behavior Change etc.) [1]. Likewise, one can begin by describing in a somewhat sparse way the determinants of clinical inertia, then try to regroup them within theoretical conceptual frameworks.

© Springer International Publishing Switzerland 2015
G. Reach, *Clinical Inertia: A Critique of Medical Reason*,
DOI 10.1007/978-3-319-09882-1_4

## Determinants of Clinical Inertia

### Initial Explanations: Denial, Exaggerated Use of "Soft Reasons" and Physician Lack of Training on the Principle of Titration

In their seminal description of the phenomenon [2], Phillips et al. had first eliminated a certain number of reasons: in particular, they rejected the idea that clinical inertia could be due to patient nonadherence, even though this reason is often put forward by physicians as a "soft reason" to not intensify treatment; neither can fear on the part of the physician of side effects of medications explain lack of titration of a treatment well tolerated up to now; neither does the cost of medications allow one to explain the clinical inertia observed when treatment is well covered; in this initial publication the authors also rejected the fact that physicians could underestimate the gravity of the situation or not be aware of guidelines. Phillips et al. therefore proposed three primary causes of clinical inertia: first, an overestimation, by physicians, of the quality of care which they dispense. Next, the use of "soft reasons", of the type: "the situation is improving", or else "in any case, the patient does not follow her diet"; finally, lack of training of physicians on the concept of titration of a treatment (intensification until a predefined target is reached). Since this initial publication, other explanations have come to enrich comprehension of the phenomenon.

### Competing Demands

We have already mentioned several times the fact that clinical inertia can occur when during an appointment the physician must deal with "another problem" other than the one which would require treatment intensification: for example, hypertension [3] or hypercholesterolemia [4] are often poorly managed when diabetes is also present, particularly when glycemia is elevated; or else, the treatment of diabetes [5] or hypertension [6] is more often intensified if it is a routine visit. In fact, Turner showed that the rate of treatment intensification for hypertension decreases with the number of comorbidities not related to it [7].

The best demonstration of this effect of "competing demands" was provided by Parchman et al., who highlighted the fact that clinical inertia is more frequent when appointments are short, and, especially, that this effect is aggravated when an intercurrent problem occurs: when appointments last between 10 and 20 min, the percentage of cases where the treatment is changed is 29 % or 66.7 % if the patient has a competing problem or not, respectively, while it is 50 and 80 % for appointments lasting over 20 min [8].

Lack of time and long patient waiting lists were recently invoked by Italian physicians as representing the major barrier to optimal management of type 2 diabetic patients at the time of diagnosis [9]. We will show in this book to what extent the issue of time is central to understanding clinical inertia.

To avoid this risk, Phillips' team proposed to adopt the following attitude during appointments: take care of the readings first (blood pressure, diabetes) before inquiring about other problems [10].

## The Effect of Uncertainty

At least regarding hypertension, uncertainty on the reality of elevated readings can be a reason – after all often justified – to not intensify treatment. As Phillips and Twombly state [10], the physician could hide behind the idea that the readings were better previously, that they are perhaps better at home due to the white coat effect (in fact, there are objective reasons to think that home blood pressure monitoring gives a better reflection of the situation than measurement in the doctor's office), or are only moderately elevated – a reason which we have mentioned several times in the previous chapter [3, 6, 11, 12]. Kerr attributed this last effect to the uncertainty in which the physician finds herself regarding the reality of poor control and the need to intervene [13]. In the study by Turner previously cited [7], treatment intensification took place more often if both systolic and diastolic blood pressure were elevated or if blood pressure was already elevated at previous visits, which is in accordance with the effect of uncertainty on clinical inertia. Redon also observed that treatment of hypertension was less often intensified when blood pressure readings were only moderately elevated, in elderly patients, or when diabetes was present [14].

To counter this effect of uncertainty, Phillips' team proposed to use the following paradigm: (1) the diagnosis of hypertension requires observation of repeated elevated readings, but (2) once the diagnosis has been pronounced, all observation of a reading above target must justify treatment, except where contraindicated [10].

## Poor Appreciation of the Actual Situation of the Patient

We have cited a study highlighting the fact that physicians were able to say if a given patient's diabetes is well or poorly controlled [15], and this is undoubtedly all the advantage of the principle of glycated hemoglobin measure, which, in a single number, allows one to compare the patient's current situation to the target one has set (familiarity with this "rating scale" undoubtedly intervenes significantly: one is considerably less at ease when this measure is uninterpretable – for example in a patient with hemochromatosis and treated by repeated therapeutic phlebotomy – and where one must base oneself on fructosamine levels).

In the case of hypertension, a study analyzed physicians' responses to an alert message triggered by the fact that recent elevated blood pressure readings had been detected by a patient computerized monitoring system; the message asked them what they had done at the time of the appointment. They answered in 27 % of cases that they did not change the treatment because "blood pressure was usually well controlled" [16]. Likewise, a Spanish study, of over 5,000 hypercholesterolemic patients showed that physicians thought that 44 % of patients were within the target defined by the National Cholesterol Education Program (NCEP ATPIII), while objectively, this was the case for only 32.8 % of them. This overestimation of good control was more often made in elderly patients, patients at high cardiovascular risk, who were physically active, or who were diabetic [17].

In fact, we will see further in this book that this causal effect of uncertainty on clinical inertia, on the one hand, or of what can be seen to a certain extent as a denial of therapeutic failure, on the other hand, must be interpreted on a much broader level.

## Characteristics of the Physician

A study carried out in 2008 in the United States specified the profile of physicians who comply more often with clinical practice guidelines: they were women, specialists (especially in gynecology and obstetrics, perhaps due to the risk of complaints), having recently completed their studies, frequently using a computer, and working in groups [18].

Interestingly enough, in this study, the effect of the date of completion of studies had no effect until 1995, which can be explained by the fact that guidelines started being disseminated in the 1990s. The effect of sex is also explained by the greater and greater feminization of the profession, over the past few years. This can suggest that the clinical inertia phenomenon should diminish with the acquisition of a "guidelines culture", a concept which should be taken into account within the very organization of medical studies.

## The Effect of Belonging to an Ethnic Minority and Being Disadvantaged

To tackle this problem, one can use the example from pediatrics, where a recent literature review made it possible to highlight a disparity, based on ethnic origin, in quality of care [19], and one can ask if this factor intervenes in the birth of clinical inertia: Cabana proposed that in the specific case of management of children's asthma, the use of guidelines could represent a means to overcome such discrimination [20].

Nevertheless, even though it is undeniable that several studies suggest that belonging to an ethnic minority or being socially disadvantaged have an impact on access to care in general and its efficiency [21–23] – a more general overview of the problem is beyond the scope of this work – their specific role in the birth of the clinical inertia phenomenon requires a nuanced interpretation: thus, regarding the management of diabetes in the United States, a study of patients enrolled in a health plan showed in fact that treatment could be intensified *more often* in case of poor control in disadvantaged patients or those belonging to an ethnic minority [24]. Likewise, a study in Israel showed that patients having a low socio-economic level were more often diabetic, managed less often to reach treatment targets, but benefitted in fact *more often* from indicators of best practice: measurement of HbA1c, microalbuminuria, performance of a dilated eye examination, insulin treatment in case of insufficient control of diabetes [25]. The study by Duru et al. did not highlight an effect of language barriers on treatment intensification in type 2 diabetic patients in case of poor control; nevertheless, low income level was clearly associated with less treatment intensification [26].

## The Doctor, Her Patient and the Health Care System

In summary, it is possible to identify many determinants of the clinical inertia phenomenon, it resulting from a certain degree of self-indulgence, for a variety of reasons, with an inadequate degree of control of chronic diseases [27, 28]. These determinants involve therefore at the same time, to paraphrase the title of the famous book by Balint devoted to "difficult" appointments, *The Doctor, His Patient and the Illness*, but also, in a major way, *the health care system*.

It is thus possible, as done by O'Connor [29] to classify the determinants of clinical inertia into three categories, depending on the physician, on the patient, or on the health care system:

1. Among the determinants depending on the physician, one finds in O'Connor's analysis first the three factors described by Phillips (overestimation of the quality of care dispensed, "soft reasons", physician lack of training on titration of treatments). O'Connor proposed to add to these explanations factors which fall under the decision making process: for example, inability by the physician to stick to a therapeutic strategy (what he calls thematic vagabonding), or on the contrary fixation on a strategy in which she feels comfortable; in summary, if the management of a chronic disease involves a process consisting of setting targets, initiating a treatment, and modifying it taking into account the level of realization of targets, clinical inertia can be due to an error, at one level or another, in this decision making process;
2. Among the factors depending on the patient, one finds the determinants of medical prescription nonadherence: denial of the disease, difficulty understanding, side effects of medications, number of medications to take, their cost, depression, addictions, poor communication between patient and physician, lack of trust in the physician;
3. Finally, among the reasons relating to the health care system, O'Connor cites for example lack of patient registries, preparation of appointments, and help in making decision. This type of classification of clinical inertia into three fields of explanations is found in qualitative studies of type 2 diabetes [30] or hypertension [31].

## Physician Clinical Inertia and Patient Nonadherence

Thus, in his classification of determinants of clinical inertia, O'Connor presents patient nonadherence, as if it were in and of itself a cause of physician clinical inertia. What's more, we have seen that Phillips himself, in physicians' "soft reasons" to not intensify treatment, cited the argument of nonadherence.

In this context, we have proposed an explanation to the fact that the two phenomena appear to go hand in hand: in fact, they have at least one reason in common, that of giving priority to the present over the future, this "clinical myopia" leading the patient to prefer the immediate and concrete reward of nonadherence, for example the pleasure of smoking a cigarette over the distant and abstract advantages of adherence with the guideline of abstaining from smoking; likewise the inert physician could prefer to avoid the immediate difficulty of a new prescription and her own fear of the occurrence of side effects over the distant and uncertain benefits that she would provide her patient by being compliant with the guideline which dictates her to intensify treatment [32]. The phenomenon of psychological insulin resistance, described in the previous chapter, is a typical example of the patient's and doctor's clinical myopia.

This synergy between physician clinical inertia and patient nonadherence is strikingly illustrated in the study by Grant which compared the behavior of physicians faced with patients that were adherent or not (the relationship was determined between the number of medication packages bought and the number of packages prescribed during the same period): in a multivariate analysis, the fact of belonging to the most adherent quartile of patients increased by 53 % the relative risk of having a treatment intensification in the 12 months that followed (95 % Confidence Interval, 1.11–1.93, p=0.01) [33].

Nevertheless, interpretation of this interaction is difficult, since it is possible that lack of treatment modification in the least adherent patients has a simple explanation: physicians prefer to direct their efforts on improving adherence. Thus, in a study of hypertensive patients, 42 % of cases of elevated blood pressure readings not having brought about treatment intensification were preceded by poor adherence, although in this study, a clear relationship between clinical inertia and nonadherence was not highlighted [34].

Thus, the determinants liable to explain the clinical inertia phenomenon appear to be many and their interactions are at times complex and difficult to interpret. This is why the construction of theoretical models is of interest, allowing for a more integrated vision.

## Theoretical Explanatory Models of Clinical Inertia

### The Knowledge-Attitude-Behavior-Result Model

As of 1999, Cabana et al. [35], based on an exhaustive study of data published at the time, attempted to answer the question: why do physicians not follow clinical practice guidelines?

They based their work on a conceptual framework defined by Woolf, describing a true "mechanism of action" of guidelines: before obtaining *a result*, in terms of morbidity, mortality, decrease in health care expenditure or efficiency of care, the guideline must first (1) lead to improved *knowledge*, on the one hand for physicians - this is done during their studies, their residency, and during continuing medical education, especially by leading them to critically assess the data from the literature - on the other hand by helping to formulate future axes of research; (2) bring about a modification of physicians' *attitudes*, led to accept new standards of care; finally (3) bring about a modification in their *behavior*, leading to their compliance with guidelines and consequently to a standardization of practices [36].

# Theoretical Explanatory Models of Clinical Inertia

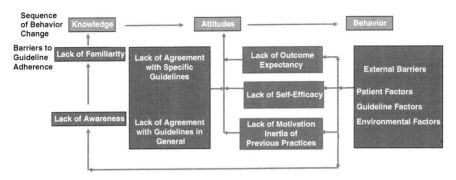

**Fig. 4.1** Barriers to guideline adherence (Modified from Ref. [35], reproduced with permission of the American Medical Association © 1999)

As Cabana [35] noted, physician behavior could have been modified without passing through a change in knowledge and attitudes, but what would be nothing but a manipulation would undoubtedly have a shorter lasting effect. It should be noted therefore that this "mechanism of action" model of guidelines, based on a modification in physician knowledge, can be referred to as cognitive. In this model, Cabana et al. were able to define seven groups of barriers, represented in Fig. 4.1, falling within the three stages of Woolf's model: knowledge, attitudes, and behavior. These authors applied this general model [35] to guidelines in the management of asthma [20, 37].

## Barriers in Knowledge

*Ignorance of guidelines:* first of all, physicians may not be aware of the very existence of guidelines, given the sum of knowledge which accumulates each day and the growing number of guidelines that have come from it. It is clear that access to medical information, through the internet, has greatly facilitated the dissemination of guidelines; on the other hand, for administrative reasons, physicians must use their computer daily. Nevertheless, lack of time can prevent physicians from getting to know guidelines in detail.

*Lack of familiarity with guidelines:* this is undoubtedly more frequent, here again due to the time needed to assimilate them. Besides, the length of guidelines can be disheartening, but summaries often exist.

## Barriers in Attitudes

*Disagreement:* the physician may in general disagree (or express reservations as we will see later) with the very principle of Evidence-Based Medicine; less often, she expresses disagreement with a specific guideline. One can sometimes reproach guidelines for becoming rapidly obsolete, especially faced with the emergence of new drug classes.

*Few results expected:* if the physician thinks that implementation of the guideline will not produce a result, she will have little tendency to implement it; for example, she can evoke patient nonadherence which would undermine the expected results of application of a guideline.

*Lack of feeling of personal effectiveness:* this is the belief that one would not be able to implement the guideline, for example due to lack of time during an appointment that is too short. The fact that patient education is not remunerated can contribute to this aspect of physician noncompliance.

*Lack of motivation, inertia:* the authors meant by this the fact that the physician is not apt to change her behavior, that she will continue to repeat what she has the habit of doing, being resistant to the idea of change and being in a way in the state of "precontemplation" in the Model of Change by Prochaska, where one considers that there is not even a problem to resolve and where one does not intend to change behavior [38].

## Barriers in Behavior

Finally, external barriers can prevent the implementation of a guideline: these may be environmental obstacles, such as lack of time, or lack of resources, or else obstacles linked to guidelines themselves (for example the existence of contradictory guidelines), and finally obstacles linked to the patient, such as difficulty to reconcile the guideline with her preferences.

As seen in Fig. 4.1, external barriers can have an impact on physician attitudes and knowledge. For example, in the management of asthma, lack of time during an appointment (external barrier) can compromise the physician's capacity (personal effectiveness, internal barrier) to present the value of a peak flow meter, and thus, lead to physician noncompliance regarding the guideline which mentions this part of patient education as being part of care.

The value of Cabana's model, by showing that the barriers to the implementation of guidelines are many, is to suggest that it suffices that only one among them be present for the guideline to not be applied. In particular, just as awareness of the prescription is not sufficient to bring about patient adherence, the fact of knowing the clinical practice guideline does not imply that it will be followed: it was therefore perfectly naive to imagine that the fact of constructing and disseminating a guideline might not be accompanied, almost automatically, by a certain degree of clinical inertia.

## The Awareness-Agreement-Adoption-Adherence Model

In 1996, Pathman et al. proposed, using vaccination as an example that compliance with a guideline passes through four stages: the physician must know the guideline, approve of it, adopt it – that is to say decide to implement it, and implement it [39]. Nevertheless, deviations from this model can exist: thus, regarding vaccination against hepatitis B, 11 % of physicians "adopted" the guideline without "approving of it", perhaps because they were affected by other forces, such as pressure from their peers, fear of lawsuits, requests by patients, obedience to current norms, etc.

In fact, the value of this model is to show that there is, stage by stage, a progressive loss of influence of the existence of a guideline on physician behavior. This was highlighted in a recent literature review of the application of this model to guidelines as diverse as drug prescriptions, prescription of home blood pressure monitoring or advising children to not watch television, with nevertheless significant variations from one guideline to another: on average, 90 % of physicians know the guideline, 70 % approve of it and adopt it, but only 40 % actually implement it [40].

Each of the four stages of this model can encounter barriers: for example, physicians may not be aware of the existence of the guideline because it was poorly disseminated, or because they do not belong to a Learned Society, or because they see few patients to which it applies. They can disagree with its content because they find it unclear, contradictory, with little applicability. They can not "adopt it" because they think they would have a hard time changing their habits, or they anticipate practical difficulties. Finally, they can not implement it due to a lack of resources, of time, because they think of the patient's knowledge and adherence.

Finally, in this study also, one could highlight deviations in relation to the model: certain physicians can agree with *the content* of a guideline without knowing it exists, or else, as Pathman demonstrated, can adopt a guideline without agreeing with it. This last point suggests that it is possible to make guidelines be adopted despite disagreement, by using incentives, for example financial, as we will see in the last part of this book.

## A Symmetrical Model Involving Physician and Patient: The Management of Dyslipidemia in Women

One can illustrate the double role of physician and patient in the birth of clinical inertia if one considers the suboptimal nature of the screening and treatment of dyslipidemia in women, by adopting the remarkable analysis conducted by Kim et al. [41].

They began by citing data from the literature showing that in certain publications (but not all) one observes that lipids are measured less often in women than in men, that, in certain randomized trials, female patients achieve control of hypercholesterolemia less often, that, in daily practice, they are prescribed less statin. To explain these disparities linked to sex, they constructed a model in which the determinants of the physician and the patient converge symmetrically to lead to clinical inertia.

In this model, patient and physician attitude play a major role: to give but two examples, women may be more concerned with the risk of breast cancer than with coronary heart disease, which explains that, within the context of "competing demands" discussed in an appointment where time is limited, measure of cholesterol or the management of hyperlipidemia is forgotten. For her part, the physician can also give priority to the screening for breast cancer, often underestimating the actual risk of coronary heart disease in women. Moreover, Kim et al. cite data suggesting that women suffer more often from disabilities, obesity, and depression, these conditions being associated with lack of screening for certain cancers or of pain management.

## Physician Guideline Compliance Model

Maue et al. constructed a model of physician compliance with guidelines [42], largely based on the Theory of Reasoned Action and the Theory of Planned Behavior proposed by Fishbein and Ajzen. Interestingly enough, these last two theories were also used to try to explain patient adherence regarding medical prescriptions [1], which shows clearly that we can conduct an identical reflection on the two issues of patient nonadherence and physician clinical inertia. Indeed, in both cases, there is *a failure to act*.

In Maue's model, and in accordance with these theories, the physician's current behavior depends on her past behavior, on her perception of her degree of control, and on her intention to apply the guideline. *Past behavior* can be assessed by asking physicians to specify how their most recent practice is in accordance with what is described in the guideline, what they think, positively or negatively, of the guideline, how they perceive the incentives to apply the guideline, which can come from colleagues, patients, or their environment. *The perception of personal control* can be assessed by asking physicians how they assess the ease or the different barriers to implementing the guideline. The result is their *intention* and their desire to implement the guideline, which, in the end is the primary determinant of their actual behavior.

An assessment of this model on about 40 physicians showed that attitude regarding guidelines and physician's perception of personal control explained two thirds of the variance in intention to use the guideline [42]. Nevertheless, this study did not make it possible to highlight a correlation between intention to use a guideline and the compliance reported by physicians or actual compliance determined by an external audit.

It is possible that this study, due to its small sample size, did not have the power needed to provide this demonstration, or else that physicians can have the intention to apply a guideline, but not do so in practice. As Mickan [40] demonstrated, the fact that one "adopts" a guideline does not necessarily mean that one puts it into practice, for reasons which we will see later.

## Another Psychological Model Applied to Comprehension of Clinical Inertia: The Regulatory Focus Theory

The Regulatory Focus Theory was developed by Higgins, based on the idea that human beings desire essentially to find pleasure and avoid pain [43]. Within this framework, we can pursue our objectives by using two types of orientations, or focuses: a promotion focus, which aims to realize accomplishments or aspirations; a prevention focus, which aims to ensure safety and responsibilities.

Both orientations have reasons: for a promotion focus, these are needs for nurturance, strong ideals, and situations involving a choice between gain and non-gain; for a prevention focus, these are needs in terms of safety, strong oughts, and situations rather seen as a choice between loss and non-loss.

They have consequences: a promotion focus leads to an awareness of the presence or absence of positive effects, and uses approach as a strategy; it is audacious and attempts to avoid errors of omission. On the contrary, a prevention focus leads to an awareness of the absence or presence of negative effects and uses avoidance as a strategy. It is cautious and attempts to avoid errors of commission.

Moreover, a promotion focus is characterized by a taking into account of a more global conception of a situation, while a prevention focus pays attention more to the details; a promotion focus is more abstract, looking to the future, a prevention focus is more concrete, looking to the present (reviewed in [44]).

Veazie and Qian [44] proposed to use this theory to explain certain aspects of clinical inertia, particularly the management of uncertainty, competing demands, and side effects of treatments. For example, given that promotion or prevention focuses aim to avoid errors of omission or of commission, respectively, a physician treating a diabetic patient and identifying with the first type of focus would have the tendency to choose a lower HbA1c intervention threshold, to avoid clinical inertia, which is itself an error of omission.

Treating a hypertensive patient, a physician within a prevention focus would be more sensitive to uncertainty of blood pressure readings, and, wanting to avoid an error of commission, would not intensify treatment.

Regarding competing demands, one can note that intensification of the management of diabetes, hypertension or hypercholesterolemia has an essentially distant objective, while a competing demand announced at the start of an appointment may seem more urgent: one understands that the physician situated within a promotion focus, more oriented towards the future, will have less risk of forgetting the treatment of chronic diseases when she is faced with an immediate competing demand on the part of the patient (recall that we ourselves had proposed to refer to the behavior of clinical inertia as "myopic" [32].)

Finally, given that promotion and prevention focuses differ in their awareness, in the first case, of a choice between gain and non-gain, and in the second, of a choice between loss and non-loss, one can understand that the first focuses the physician's attention on the advantages of treatment and the second on the inconveniences of its side effects. In summary, this analysis suggests that the avoidance of pain which characterizes a prevention focus could be conceptually associated with clinical inertia.

Incidentally, the fact that promotion and prevention focuses are linked to abstract and distant concepts, and concrete and immediate concepts, respectively, is consistent with the categorization of concepts as high and low level in the construal level theory proposed by Trope and Liberman, which proposes that we have the tendency to categorize concepts into two types: those of high-level, abstract and oriented towards the future, and those of low-level, concrete and based on the immediate; for example, if one thinks of reading on an abstract level, one will think that it enriches the mind; if one thinks of it on a concrete level, one will mention the book that one is reading [45]. We ourselves had proposed to use this last theory as an explanatory conceptual framework of patient nonadherence [46]. This shows again to what extent the two phenomena of physician clinical inertia and patient nonadherence are, also from a theoretical point of view, linked.

\*

\*\*

In this chapter it has bit by bit emerged that the reasons for the physician to not follow guidelines which she is aware of and even that she approves of are in fact numerous. In other words, it may even be *rational* for the physician to have a behavior that, strictly speaking, in light of a medicine which advocates the existence of guidelines to guide medical practice, one can refer to as clinical inertia.

Yet, guidelines are likewise based on *a rationale* and at times on what one calls, in Evidence-Based Medicine terminology, a high level of evidence. There seems therefore to be a contradiction between two dynamics. To ask how clinical inertia is possible, and if it is not in fact but an expression of this contradiction, leads one therefore to examine in more detail the very principles of Evidence-Based Medicine and physicians' reactions to its advent.

## References

1. Reach G. The mental mechanisms of patient adherence to long term therapies, mind and care, foreword by Pascal Engel, "Philosophy and Medicine" series, Springer, forthcoming.
2. Phillips LS, Branch WT, Cook CB, Doyle JP, El-Kebbi IM, Gallina DL, Miller CD, Ziemer DC, Barnes CS. Clinical inertia. Ann Intern Med. 2001;135:825–34.
3. Bolen SD, Samuels TA, Yeh HC, Marnopoulos SS, McGuire M, Abuid M, Brancati FL. Failure to intensify antihypertensive treatment by primary care providers: a cohort study in adults with diabetes mellitus and hypertension. J Gen Intern Med. 2008;23:543–50.
4. Willig JH, Jacson DA, Westfall AO, Allison J, Chang PW, Raper J, Saag MS, Mugavero MJ. Clinical inertia in the management of low-density lipoprotein abnormalities in an HIV clinic. Clin Infect Dis. 2008;46:1315–8.
5. Bolen SD, Bricker E, Samuels TA, Yeh HC, Marinopoulos SS, McGuire M, Abuid M, Brancati FL. Factors associated with intensification of oral diabetes medications in primary care provider-patient dyads: a cohort study. Diabetes Care. 2009;32:25–31.
6. Viera AJ, Schmid D, Bostrom S, Yow A, Lawrence W, DuBard CA. Level of blood pressure above goal and clinical inertia in a Medicaid population. J Am Soc Hypertens. 2010;4:244–54.
7. Turner BJ, Hollenbeak CS, Weiner M, Ten Have T, Tang SS. Effect of unrelated comorbid conditions on hypertension management. Ann Intern Med. 2008;148:578–86.
8. Parchman ML, Pugh JA, Romero RL, Bowers KW. Competing demands or clinical inertia: the case of elevated glycosylated hemoglobin. Ann Fam Med. 2007;5:196–201.
9. Suraci C, Mulas F, Rossi MC, Gentile S, Giorda CB. Management of newly diagnosed patients with type 2 diabetes: what are the attitudes of physicians? A SUBITO!AMD survey on the early diabetes treatment in Italy. Acta Diabetol. 2012;49:429–33.
10. Phillips LS, Twombly JG. It's time to overcome clinical inertia. Ann Intern Med. 2008;148:783–5.
11. Andrade SE, Gurwitz JH, Field TS, Kelleher M, Majumdar SR, Reed G, Black R. Hypertension management: the care gap between clinical guidelines and clinical practice. Am J Manag Care. 2004;10:481–6.
12. Gil-Guillén V, Orozco-Beltran D, Pérez RP, Alfonso JL, Redon J, Pertusa-Martinez S, Navarro J, Cea-Calvo L, Quirce-Andres F, Merino-Sanchez J, Carratala C, Martin-Moreno JM. Clinical inertia in diagnosis and treatment of hypertension in primary care: quantification and association factors. Blood Press. 2010;19:3–10.
13. Kerr EA, Zikmund-Fisher BJ, Klamerus ML, Subramanian U, Hogan MM, Hofer TP. The role of clinical uncertainty in treatment decisions for diabetic patients with uncontrolled blood pressure. Ann Intern Med. 2008;148:717–27.
14. Redón J, Coca A, Lázaro P, Aguilar MD, Cabañas M, Gil N, Sánchez-Zamorano MA, Aranda P. Factors associated with therapeutic inertia in hypertension: validation of a predictive model. J Hypertens. 2010;28:1770–7.

15. El-Kebbi IM, Ziemer DC, Musey VC, Gallina DL, Bernard AM, Phillips LS. Diabetes in urban African-Americans. IX Provider adherence to management protocols. Diabetes Care. 1997;20:698–703.
16. Rose AJ, Shimada SL, Rothendler JA, Reisman JI, Glassman PA, Berlowitz DR, Kressin NR. The accuracy of clinician perceptions of "usual" blood pressure control. J Gen Intern Med. 2008;23:180–3.
17. Banegas JR, Vegazo O, Serrano P, Luengo E, Mantilla T, Fernández R, Civeira F, HISPALIPID Study Group Investigators. The gap between dyslipidemia control perceived by physicians and objective control patterns in Spain. Atherosclerosis. 2006;188:420–4.
18. Sammer CE, Lykens K, Singh KP. Physician characteristics and the reported effect of evidence-based practice guidelines. Health Serv Res. 2008;43:569–81.
19. Flores G. Technical report–racial and ethnic disparities in the health and health care of children. Pediatrics. 2010;125:e979–1020.
20. Cabana MD, Flores G. The role of clinical practice guidelines in enhancing quality and reducing racial/ethnic disparities in paediatrics. Paediatr Respir Rev. 2002;3:52–8.
21. Verma A, Birger R, Bhatt H, Murray J, Millett C, Saxena S, Banarsee R, Gnani S, Majeed A. Ethnic disparities in diabetes management: a 10-year population-based repeated cross-sectional study in UK primary care. J Public Health (Oxf). 2010;32:250–8.
22. McLean G, Guthrie B, Sutton M. Differences in the quality of primary medical care for CVD and diabetes across the NHS: evidence from the quality and outcomes framework. BMC Health Serv Res. 2007;7:74.
23. Tseng CW, Tierney EF, Gerzoff RB, Dudley RA, Waitzfelder B, Ackermann RT, Karter AJ, Piette J, Crosson JC, Ngo-Metzger Q, Chung R, Mangione CM. Race/ethnicity and economic differences in cost-related medication underuse among insured adults with diabetes: the Translating Research into Action for Diabetes study. Diabetes Care. 2008;31:261–6.
24. Brown AF, Gregg EW, Stevens MR, Karter AJ, Weinberger M, Safford MM, Gary TL, Caputo DA, Waitzfelder B, Kim C, Beckles GL. Race, ethnicity, socioeconomic position, and quality of care for adults with diabetes enrolled in managed care: the Translating Research Into Action for Diabetes (TRIAD) study. Diabetes Care. 2005;28:2864–70.
25. Jotkowitz AB, Rabinowitz G, Raskin Segal A, Weitzman R, Epstein L, Porath A. Do patients with diabetes and low socioeconomic status receive less care and have worse outcomes? A national study. Am J Med. 2006;119:665–9.
26. Duru OK, Bilik D, McEwen LN, Brown AF, Karter AJ, Curb JD, Marrero DG, Lu SE, Rodriguez M, Mangione CM. Primary language, income and the intensification of anti-glycemic medications in managed care: the (TRIAD) study. J Gen Intern Med. 2011;26:505–11.
27. Faria C, Wenzel M, Lee KW, Coderre K, Nichols J, Belletti DA. A narrative review of clinical inertia: focus on hypertension. J Am Soc Hypertens. 2009;3:267–76.
28. Triplitt C. Improving treatment success rates for type 2 diabetes: recommendations for a changing environment. Am J Manag Care. 2010;16:S195–200.
29. O'Connor PJ, Sperl-Hillen JAM, Johnson PE, Rush WA, Biltz G. Clinical inertia and outpatient medical errors. In: Henriksen K, Battles JB, Marks ES, Lewin DI, editors. Advances in patient safety: from research to implementation, vol 2: Concepts and methodology. Rockville: Agency for Healthcare Research and Quality (US), 2005.
30. Brown JB, Harris SB, Webster-Bogaert S, Wetmore S, Faulds C, Stewart M. The role of patient, physician and systemic factors in the management of type 2 diabetes mellitus. Fam Pract. 2002;19:344–9.
31. Howes F, Hansen E, Williams D, Nelson M. Barriers to diagnosing and managing hypertension – a qualitative study in Australian general practice. Aust Fam Physician. 2010;39:511–6.
32. Reach G. Patient nonadherence and healthcare-provider inertia are clinical myopia. Diabetes Metab. 2008;34:382–5.
33. Grant R, Adams AS, Trinacty CM, Zhang F, Kleinman K, Soumerai SB, Meigs JB, Ross-Degnan D. Relationship between patient medication adherence and subsequent clinical inertia in type 2 diabetes glycemic management. Diabetes Care. 2007;30:807–12.
34. Heisler M, Hogan MM, Hofer TP, Schmittdiel JA, Pladevall M, Kerr EA. When more is not better: treatment intensification among hypertensive patients with poor medication adherence. Circulation. 2008;117:2884–92.

35. Cabana MD, Rand CS, Powe NR, Wu AW, Wilson MH, Abboud P-AC, Rubin HR. Why don't physicians follow clinical practice guidelines? A framework for improvement. JAMA. 1999;282:1458–67.
36. Woolf SH. Practice guidelines: a new reality in medicine, III: impact on patient care. Arch Intern Med. 1993;153:2646–55.
37. Cabana MD, Ebel BE, Cooper-Patrick L, Powe NR, Rubin HR, Rand CS. Barriers pediatricians face when using asthma guidelines. Arch Pediatr Adolesce Med. 2000;154:683–93.
38. Main DS, Cohen SJ, DiClemente CC. Measuring physician readiness to change cancer screening: preliminary results. Am J Prev Med. 1995;11:54–8.
39. Pathman DE, Konrad TR, Freed GL, Freeman VA, Koch GG. The awareness-to-adherence model of the steps to clinical guideline compliance: the case of pediatric vaccine recommendations. Med Care. 1996;34:873–89.
40. Mickan S, Burls A, Glasziou P. Patterns of 'leakage' in the utilisation of clinical guidelines: a systematic review. Postgrad Med J. 2011;87:670–9.
41. Kim C, Hofer T, Kerr EA. Review of evidence and explanations for suboptimal screening and treatment of dyslipiemia in women. A conceptual model. J Gen Intern Med. 2003;18:854–63.
42. Maue SK, Segal R, Kimberlin CL, Lipowski EE. Predicting physician guideline compliance: an assessment of motivators and perceived barriers. Am J Manag Care. 2004;10:383–91.
43. Higgins ET. Beyond pleasure and pain. Am Psychol. 1997;52:1280–300.
44. Veazie PJ, Qian F. A role for regulatory focus in explaining and combating clinical inertia. J Eval Clin Pract. 2011;17:1147–52.
45. Trope Y, Liberman N. Temporal construal. Psychol Rev. 2003;110:403–21.
46. Reach G. Obstacles to patient education in chronic diseases: a trans-theoretical analysis. Patient Educ Couns. 2009;77:192–6.

# The Physician and Evidence-Based Medicine

**5**

### Abstract

This chapter analyzes the principle of Evidence-Based Medicine which was initially aimed at making it so that patients benefit from the best available treatments. Thus Evidence-Based Medicine is supposed to help the physician make decisions in a fundamentally uncertain context, both at the level of diagnosis and of therapeutic choices. However, as the founders of Evidence-Based Medicine repeated time and again, medical decisions should not only rely on science, but also on the characteristics and the wishes of the patient. The second part of the chapter presents a critique of Evidence-Based Medicine, in three parts: (1) What physicians think about it, (2) Methodological criticisms, in particular those concerning the principle of randomized clinical trials, (3) Finally an epistemological criticism, inspired by the work of Donald Schön, *The Reflective Practitioner*: Evidence-Based Medicine relies on a Technical Rationality which allows one to solve problems, while the real difficulty for physicians in their daily practice is not to solve problems, but to formulate them. Rather than a Technical Rationality, they call upon more complex decision-making processes relying on their experience.

## A New Way to Practice Medicine

It is said that one can trace the beginnings of the concept of Evidence-Based Medicine to the start of the nineteenth century, precisely to the work by the English physician Thomas Beddoe who demanded in 1808 in "A Letter to the Right Honourable Sir Joseph Banks ... on the causes and removal of the prevailing discontents, imperfections, and abuses in medicine" a collection, an archiving and a sharing of evidence within a "national bank of medical wealth, where each individual practitioner may deposit his grains of knowledge, and draw out, in return, the stock, accumulated by all his brethren." One cites also the importance of the trial, published in

© Springer International Publishing Switzerland 2015
G. Reach, *Clinical Inertia: A Critique of Medical Reason*,
DOI 10.1007/978-3-319-09882-1_5

1834 by Pierre Charles Alexandre Louis, showing that it is possible to prove the ineffectiveness of bloodletting [1].

But one must await the critique formulated in the 1970s by Cochrane (1909–1988) regarding the fact that only 10–25 % of medical decisions are based on established scientific evidence [2] before a few years later, in 1992, the term *Evidence-Based Medicine* is forged by Guyatt et al. [3].

## Objectives of Evidence-Based Medicine

In the mind of its founders, the purpose of Evidence-Based Medicine was to put an end, through an educational approach, to the disparities in treatments which make it that certain patients do not benefit from the best medicine available. It's about "integrating individual clinical expertise and the best external evidence." This can only be obtained through systematic research which assesses the quality of available information and classifies it according to a level of proof, taking into account the type of study which led to its collection. Nevertheless, in no instance can "evidence" replace the physician's judgment or experience: Evidence-Based Medicine completes traditional medical practice but does not replace it. Finally, one can see the practice of Evidence-Based Medicine as the integration of three components: the Evidence, the physician's clinical experience and the preferences of the patient regarding care [4, 5].

## Data and Guidelines: Different Levels of Evidence

It is generally considered that the "highest level of evidence" comes from Randomized Clinical Trials (RCT): experimental studies where patients selected for a treatment intervention, for example, are divided randomly ("randomized") for instance in two groups, the first receiving a treatment (T), the second in general a placebo or another treatment to which one wishes to compare the treatment (T). A high level of evidence is also obtained based on "meta-analyses" which consist of analyzing according to a rigorous methodology the results of comparable studies, in particular showing that an effect can be observed in several centers. Needless to say, there is also a high level of evidence when the treatment brings about an obvious improvement ("all or nothing" situations, for example when one has established that all patients died before introduction of a treatment and that now some survive due to the treatment, or when some patients died before introduction of a treatment and that now all survive due to the treatment) [5]. One gives humorously the use of a parachute as the type of situation of all or nothing in which the carrying out of larger randomized clinical trials would be questionable! [6].

Obviously, the level of evidence is lower when one considers retrospective publications comparing series of patients having and patients free from a disease ("case-control studies"). Four levels of evidence are often defined. Clinical practice guidelines are constructed based on the level of evidence provided by the available

# A New Way to Practice Medicine

| Level of scientific evidence produced by the literature (therapeutic studies) | Guideline Grade |
|---|---|
| **Level 1**<br>• High power randomized controlled trials<br>• Meta-analysis of randomized controlled trials<br>• Analysis of decision based on well conducted trials | **A**<br>Established scientific evidence |
| **Level 2**<br>• Low power randomized controlled trials<br>• Well conducted non-randomized controlled studies<br>• Cohort studies | **B**<br>Scientific presumption |
| **Level 3**<br>• Case-control studies<br><br>**Level 4**<br>• Controlled studies with significant biases<br>• Retrospective studies<br>• Case series studies | **C**<br>Low level of evidence |

**Table 5.1** Level of scientific evidence provided by the literature (therapeutic studies), and grade of guidelines derived from it (Translated from Haute Autorité de Santé [7])

studies. They have therefore, likewise, a variable level of proof, going from "established scientific proof" to "scientific presumption" and "low level of evidence". Table 5.1 represents the different levels of evidence and the grade of guidelines used by the French Haute Autorité de Santé [7].

## What Is Not Evidence-Based Medicine

Given that Evidence-Based Medicine is an integration of three components, the Evidence, the physician's clinical experience and the preferences of the patient regarding care, it represents a "bottom-up" process and could in no way lead to development of medical conduct which would come down to the servile application of "cookbooks": thus, "external clinical evidence can inform, but can never replace, individual clinical expertise, and it is this expertise that decides whether the external evidence applies to the individual patient at all and, if so, how it should be integrated into a clinical decision. Similarly, any external guideline must be integrated with individual clinical expertise in deciding whether and how it matches the patient's clinical state, predicament, and preferences, and thus whether it should be applied" [4].

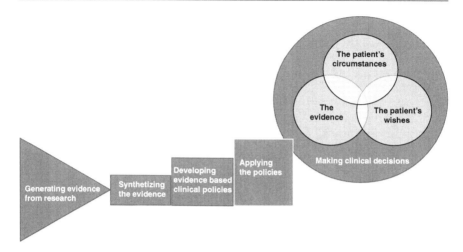

**Fig. 5.1** The path from the generation of evidence to the application of evidence (From Ref. [8], Reproduced with permission from BMJ Publishing Group Ltd.)

## Evidence-Based Medicine: Clinical Practice Assisted by the Development of Clinical Practice Guidelines

### Clinical Practice in the Context of Evidence-Based Medicine

In this new state of mind, the physician confronted with a particular clinical situation and asking herself which is the best diagnostic (should she prescribe such and such lab test?) or therapeutic (which is the best treatment to offer?) choice uses a process that passes through four stages: (1) transform the need for information regarding a given patient into a question formulated in a clear and precise way; (2) search as effectively as possible in the medical literature for the most relevant articles; (3) critically assess the validity (trustworthiness) and the value (applicability) of results contained in these articles and extract the Evidence on which to base clinical decisions (diagnostic or therapeutic); (4) deduce the measures to be taken for the patient being considered [5]. Next, it's a matter of implementing them.

Obviously, the first stage of the process, the way of asking the question, is crucial and is itself based on a decomposition into stages, described by the **PICO** method: what is the characteristic of the **P**atient or the **P**roblem, what **I**ntervention is one considering, what will be the **C**omparison, what will be the **O**utcome which will constitute the judgment criterion?

### Clinical Practice Guidelines, Assistance in Medical Decisions in the Evidence-Based Medicine State of Mind

*In the beginning there was the Evidence*: Fig. 5.1 represents the path that goes from creation of evidence to its application within clinical practice [8].

The first stage is therefore the production of Evidence, based on scientific research. The authors of this figure deliberately represented this first phase in the form of a wedge, based on a large research base "up-front" to arrive at the small number of clinical trials which will provide the end demonstration that such and such new diagnostic test or such and such new treatment is beneficial. As noted by Haynes and Haines [8], there are many more studies that do not make it to the apex of the wedge, but which enter into competition with the actually useful data in the mind of readers of the medical literature: the mixture within the same Journals of articles demonstrating, for example by a large randomized trial, the effectiveness of a treatment (communication from researchers to physicians) and articles describing preliminary data (communication between researchers) impedes clinicians, through an excess of information, in having access to useful information [9].

Next there is the synthesis of evidence, and this is truly a *synthesis*, that is to say the stage which follows *the analysis* of scientific data. Yet there are two obstacles to the practical carrying out of this essential stage: first, the immensity of data available, the difficulty of finding the relevant data – although this difficulty is remarkably resolved by modern access to databases (older clinicians remember the era before the internet and *PubMed*, their weekly reading of *Current Contents*, and their dependence on librarians!); next there is the difficulty of performing a true critical analysis of this data – although methodologies of critical analysis of articles have been disseminated, and, what's more, assessment of medical students' abilities in this specific field is an integral part of the testing of their knowledge – and finally the stage of synthesis itself. This is the value of Journals which edit critical syntheses, sparing the individual clinician a task for which she would have neither the practical possibility, nor the actual aptitude, nor the time needed. One can within this framework cite the *Cochrane Library*, which publishes syntheses on most large clinical questions [10].

The following stage is that of the development of clinical practice guidelines. It is carried out by groups of experts at a national or international level. It is important that these guidelines actually take into account all the available data, its level of evidence, the different aspects of therapeutic strategies, from their effectiveness to the consequences on the Quality of Life of patients, to the economic impact, and the resources necessary etc., and the local context in which they could be applied, since they will lead to the development of true care policies. As emphasized by Haynes and Haines, the development of clinical practice guidelines represents the most difficult stage in the path leading from research data to its practical implementation [8]. There exist precise rules on the way to develop clinical practice guidelines (guidelines on guidelines), and it is desirable that physicians who will use these guidelines are aware of this methodology, at least broadly [7].

Finally, there is the practical application of Evidence-Based Health Care policies. These must pass essentially through two stages: firstly, the dissemination of guidelines and, if necessary, the transformation of the health care system in order to allow it to implement guidelines in practice, if, for example, these require certain resources which are not available; secondly, their application. As seen in Fig. 5.1, this decision comes back to the physician. In the best practice of Evidence-Based Medicine, she would combine three elements to make her decision: the Evidence itself, but also the characteristics of the patient, with the major question being to know if this singular patient falls under the guideline in question, finally, the preferences of the patient.

This last remark emphasizes the need for training of medical students and physicians in the concepts of Evidence-Based Medicine. Particular emphasis should be placed on critical analysis of guidelines themselves; physicians must learn to choose a "good" guideline, know how to answer questions such as "is the guideline valid?", with the crucial question, as stated – "does it apply to the patient I have in front of me?" [11] Regarding teaching, the founders of the Evidence-Based Medicine movement, rightly insist upon what one must not do [12]: the worst would be "when learning how to do research is emphasized over how to use it; when learning how to do statistics is emphasized over how to interpret them; when teaching EBM is limited only to finding flaws in published research; when teaching portrays EBM as substituting research evidence for, rather than adding it to, clinical expertise, patient values, and circumstances [...]; when it humiliates learners for not already knowing the "right" fact or answer; when it bullies learners to decide or act based on fear of others' authority or power, rather than on authoritative evidence and rational argument."

## Evidence-Based Medicine, Medicine Practiced Within a Context of Uncertainty

As seen in Table. 5.1, Evidence is established with variable levels of evidence, and the same is true of the guidelines derived from it. Indeed, Evidence has essentially a statistical nature: the occurrence of an event has a certain *probability*, which is in general *never completely* equal to 1 (it is *certain* that the event will occur), or to 0 (it is *certain* that it will not occur). One is therefore never *entirely sure* in theory that the patient has the disease one thinks she has, and when one performs a diagnostic test, it can decrease the degree of uncertainty, but cannot abolish it entirely; likewise, when one gives a treatment, one can *never* be *entirely sure* that the effect will be beneficial or that there won't be side effects, and results from studies tell us only, *statistically*, that, for example, within the population which was studied in such and such large randomized clinical trial, patients who received the active medication died less often 1 year after a first infarction than those who received the placebo (but there were nevertheless deaths within the group of patients treated by the active molecule and survivors within the placebo group).

It is precisely the fact that the physician works within a context of uncertainty which constitutes the reason for being of Evidence-Based Medicine: as Kamhi wrote recently [13], uncertainty is one of the pre-conditions of Evidence-Based Medicine, because to search for the evidence of what one knows already is contrary to the basic tenets of Evidence-Based Medicine. This is what emerges when one examines in more detail the two situations of diagnosis and therapy.

### Uncertainty Within the Field of Diagnosis

Let's take first the value of a diagnostic test for a given disease. What Evidence-Based Medicine provides, is a quantification of the fact that its results are almost never *entirely* conclusive (Fig. 5.2): for example, it will be positive in 85 % of cases

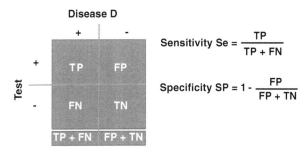

**Fig. 5.2** Sensitivity and specificity of a diagnostic test

in patients with the disease ("True Positives", TP) but it will therefore be negative in 15 % of these patients ("False Negatives", FN). It will be negative in 90 % of individuals free from the disease ("True Negatives", TN), but it will be positive in 10 % of individuals without the disease ("False Positives", FP). One can thus define the *sensitivity* of the test, that is to say the *probability* of having a positive test result if the individual has the disease, which is equal to TP/(TP+FN), in this example, 85 %, and the *specificity* of the test, that is to say the probability that the test be negative in individuals free from the disease, which is equal to TN/(FP+TN), or 1 − FP/(FP+TN), in this example 90 %.

Thus, there is uncertainty in that a diagnosis is not necessarily confirmed, simply because the result of a test is positive, and it is not eliminated simply because the result is negative. Nevertheless, the attributes of the test, its sensitivity and its specificity, have a significant effect on the way *in which what we think approaches reality* (the patient does or does not have the disease): this is why it is good that, on the one hand, the sensitivity be very elevated - in this case, a negative result contributes to eliminate the diagnosis, and that, on the other hand, its specificity be very elevated – a positive result reinforces the diagnosis.

This is in fact the goal of all diagnostic tests (the term being considered very generally – this could be a question one asks the patient, a bioassay, an x-ray examination etc.): to modify, in the mind of the physician, the degree of conviction in what she thinks; if, before asking the question I think *in theory* that something (for example, the patient has a disease D) has a certain probability $p(D)$, this is transformed into a "post-test" probability when I receive the answer, for example that the test is positive. This introduces the notion of *conditional probability*, which can be noted, if the test is positive, as $p(D/+)$.

## Bayes' Theorem

*Bayes' theorem*, coming from an essay written by the reverend Thomas Bayes (1702–1761) and published posthumously in 1763 under the title "An Essay towards solving a Problem in the Doctrine of Chances" [14], allows one to, *in a theoretical way*, quantify this modification. The degree of certainty post-test – or what remains of uncertainty – depends not only on the value of the test, its sensitivity and its specificity, but also on the probability *in theory*, that is the pre-test probability, which was that which existed before one conducted the test and knew the result:

according to Laplace's formulation of Bayes' theorem, the relationship between post-test probability, pre-test probability, and the attributes of the test (sensitivity and specificity) can be described as follows:

$p(D)$: pre-test probability of having the disease
$p(D/+)$: post-test probability of having the disease if the test is positive

$$p(D/+) = \frac{p(D) \times \text{Se}}{p(D) \times \text{Se} + \left[1 - p(D)\right] \times (1 - \text{Sp})}$$

$p(D/-)$: post-test probability of having the disease if the test is negative

$$p(D/-) = \frac{p(D) \times (1 - \text{Se})}{p(D) \times (1 - \text{Se}) + \left[1 - p(D)\right] \times \text{Sp}}$$

where Se and Sp refer to the sensitivity and specificity of the test, respectively.

These formulas give the curves represented in Fig. 5.3, where the post-test probability is represented as a function of the pre-test probability, in the case of a sensitivity of 0.80 and specificity of 0.70 (test 1), and of a sensitivity of 0.90 and specificity of 0.70 (test 2), when the response of the tests is positive (upper curves), or negative (lower curves).

What does a clinical trial aiming to assess a test do? It consists, within a population of patients, on the one hand of giving the attributes of the test, that is to say its sensitivity and specificity; on the other hand, by giving the pre-test probability, it provides an indication on the prevalence of the disease on which the test is used: this data can therefore help the clinician to assess - in fact by using Bayes' theorem more or less explicitly – what she can expect to gain or to lose in degree of certainty that the patient has the disease.

It is important to note that the gain of conviction if the test is positive and the loss of conviction if it is negative depend closely on the pre-test probability. Indeed, as seen in Fig. 5.3, if one starts with a pre-test probability of 70 %, as is the case in this figure, in the case of a test having a sensitivity of 0.80 and specificity of 0.70 (test 1), the post-test probability would be 86 % if the test is positive and 40 % if it is negative. The changes are shown by the vertical arrows. If one is almost entirely sure that the patient does not have (on the left) or has (on the right), the disease, one sees that the results of the test would modify little the probability, and performing this test is of little use. One sees thus how the type of data provided by the scientific evaluation of diagnostic tests (Evidence-Based Medicine) and Bayesian type reasoning can help the physician to make her decision: how knowledge of the characteristics of a test will help her decide (i) if there is a need to implement it and (ii) if its result would modify her therapeutic decision.

The second stage of the process depends in fact not only on the post-test probability, but also on the intervention threshold that the physician has set herself: in a Bayesian type process, the clinician will use two probability thresholds, the treatment threshold and the test threshold [15].

# A New Way to Practice Medicine

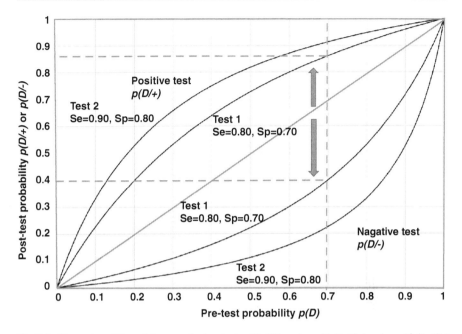

**Fig. 5.3** Illustration of Bayes' theorem, for two tests with different sensitivity (Se) and specificity (Sp)

1. *The treatment threshold*: if the pre-test probability is above this threshold, it is already so likely that the patient has the disease that I do not need a test to begin treatment. If I had to absolutely confirm my hypothesis, for example due to the side effects of the treatment, I would use a test with a high specificity, in order to disprove my diagnosis if it were negative. And if this were the case, I should then perform an additional test, and choose the test considered as the "gold standard", to avoid having missed the diagnosis of the disease based on a falsely negative result.
2. *The test threshold*: a pre-test probability below this threshold suggests that it is so improbable *in theory* that the patient has the disease that there isn't even a need to perform the test (even if it were positive, I would not consider treating the patient). If, in this case, I had to absolutely confirm this hypothesis, for example due to the gravity of the disease if it is not treated, I would use a test with a high sensitivity: if it is negative, this would mean that it is truly almost certain that the patient does not have the disease. But if it were positive, one must then perform another test, by using again the test considered as the "gold standard" to avoid treating a person based on a falsely positive result of the initial test.

Therefore the question is asked particularly when the initial pre-test probability is situated within an intermediate zone, between the test threshold (I must perform the test) and the treatment threshold. That's the value of Bayes' theorem: it allows one to say if the expected post-test probability, given the initial probability and the characteristics of the test (sensitivity and specificity) will exceed the treatment threshold – one must treat, or will remain within an intermediate zone – one must perform another test, or will drop, because the result was negative, below the test threshold; in which case, one can stop the investigations.

Nevertheless, one notes that this type of calculation is essentially based on estimations of test characteristics (sensitivity, specificity) and the pre-test probability coming from assessments which were performed. Is it legitimate to apply them to the patient the physician is faced with? Is this patient identical, or sufficiently similar, to the patients in the study which made this assessment possible? One understands here immediately the value of meta-analyses, since in this case, one bases oneself on the results of several studies. Moreover, what is the degree of trust that the physician can have regarding the study which made it possible to obtain these estimations?

## Uncertainty Within the Therapeutic Field

Needless to say, in the decision to treat, one does not take into account only the probability that the patient does or does not have the disease whose diagnosis leads to the treatment. One must also consider the effect of the treatment. Let's use as example a disease complicated by a coronary event whose rate of occurrence was specified, in a study, as being 6 % during treatment with placebo (Control Event Rate = CER). Within the group of patients treated with the active molecule, the event rate was only 4.5 % (Experimental Event Rate EER). One can say that the "Relative Risk Reduction" RRR was (CER − EER)/CER = 25 %. The Absolute Risk Reduction ARR would be CER − EER = 1.5 %. The Number Needed to Treat NNT to avoid an event would be 1/ARR = 66 patients. Here is another situation, in which the risk of occurrence of an event decreases from a CER of 25 % to an EER of 5 %: the calculation gives an ARR of 20 % and an NNT of 4 needed to treat to avoid an event. Undoubtedly, in the second situation, the physician will be more inclined to start treatment.

But, again, this data is essentially statistical, based on a cohort of patients leading to the concept of "average patient". Uncertainty will necessarily remain: again, is the patient that the physician is faced with similar to the "average patients" in the study? Will she take her treatment? What would have been the number needed to treat if in the study one had in the inclusion period not excluded, as is often done, nonadherent patients etc. And again, can one trust the study or studies which have shown all this?

## Quantitative Formalization of Patient Preferences

It is therefore possible to assess the modification of risk that the patient is exposed to, provided by the implementation of a treatment, and to present to her the results of this analysis. Nevertheless, her decision will not only take into account this probability. It will also consider the consequences of what would occur, in the case where the treatment is implemented or in the case where it is not, for her well-being, for her quality of life, for what one can call more generally her state of health. In this way she could assess her "preference" between several options.

In this field also, it is possible to give a quantitative formalization of this preference: economists call "utility" the measurement of the preference given to the state of health obtained after a treatment, and it is usually expressed as a decimal value between zero and 1, for example 0.4: the value 1 typically represents a perfect state of health, and the value zero represents death. One can what's more have a negative value if the patient imagines that a consequence of an intervention would be worse than death [16].

It therefore becomes possible to construct a "decision tree", describing the consequences of different treatment strategies and their consequences. Let's take the case of a disease where the question is whether or not to implement an innovative treatment T, for example thrombolytic therapy after an acute stroke (Fig. 5.4).

By convention, the moment (the "node") where one has to make a decision between several therapeutic options is represented by a square; the consequence of an option is random: an option therefore leads to a "probability node" represented by a circle; in fact several events can occur, situated at the end of each arm coming from this circle, and represented by triangles (stationary nodes). One can therefore calculate for each of these events an "expected utility" by multiplying the value of the "utility", seen above, by the probability of occurrence of the event.

In the example in Fig. 5.4, the treatment T can cure the disease, but has a mortality rate of 5 %. If one does not implement it, the patient will definitely (probability $P = 1$) be left with a chronic disability from her disease to which she attributes a value, called above "utility", of $U_x$, for example of 0.8 (which would mean that she considers that living with the residual disability gives her a quality of life 0.8 times the quality of normal life, let's say that her quality of life with the disability is amputated by 20 %). However, if one implements treatment T, one arrives at a probability node leading to two types of events: with a probability $P_d$, of death ("utility"$=0$), or, with a probability $(1 - P_d)$, of being cured ("utility"$= 1$).

One can calculate an "expected utility" for each of the two therapeutic options. The expected utility of standard therapy is $1 \times U_x$, in this example $1 \times 0.8 = 0.8$. That of treatment T is calculated by adding together the expected utilities of each of the possible results: that of death, $P_d \times 0$, to which one adds that of being cured, $(1 - P_d) \times 1$. If one knows, according to studies, that the rate of treatment failure, which leads to death, is 5 %, the calculation gives for this arm of the decision tree a value of $0.05 \times 0 + 0.95 \times 1 = 0.95$, which is greater than 0.80. *According to this statistical reasoning*, it is therefore in the patient's best interest to try the new treatment.

This is of course a very simplified diagram: for example, the treatment itself may not have but two results, life or death; it can have temporary or definitive side effects, and it will therefore be a matter, for the patient, of quantifying in the form of a "utility" the value that she gives to her life with these side effects. Neither must one underestimate the difficulty, for the patient, to quantify the "utility" of a situation, represented in Fig. 5.4 under the term $U_x$. Methods were proposed for this, especially by asking the patient to consider the dilemma in the form of a bet, or more simply, by using a visual analogue scale [17].

At the end of this overview of the principles of Evidence-Based Medicine, it indeed emerges that its development and its translation in the form of clinical practice guidelines can represent an aid in medical decisions within a context of uncertainty, itself linked to the variability of living phenomena. One therefore notes that

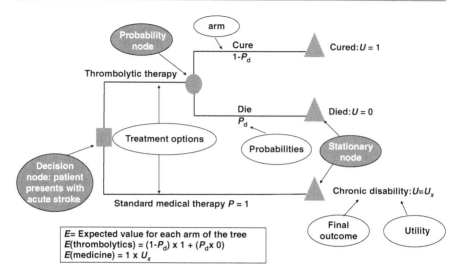

**Fig. 5.4** An example of a decision tree (From Mayer [15], Reproduced with permission of Cambridge University Press)

Evidence-Based Medicine was proposed at first with the intention of limiting the variability of medical practices. But it itself encounters another variability, that of living phenomena, and the method it has developed was chosen to answer to this variability: if it uses randomized clinical trials, it is because they are the only method which allows one to limit as much as possible the effect of the noise from the signal that one wishes to detect. Next, it teaches practitioners to use this *evidence*: therapeutic choices are presented in the form of decision trees which take into account the probabilities associated with each alternative, that is to say the variability, such as it has been quantified. Finally, it disseminates the measures to be taken in the form of guidelines: it hopes thus to limit the variability of medical practices, which is its initial objective.

## Evidence-Based Medicine: A Change of Paradigm?

Thomas Kuhn described the evolution of scientific theories in the form of changes of paradigm: a scientific paradigm can be described as the prevailing conceptual framework in which discoveries are made, up until the moment where new discoveries can no longer adapt to current theories. A change of paradigm then takes place [18]. One can ask if the emergence of Evidence-Based Medicine actually represents a change of paradigm in medicine. As noted by Howick [19], this new science at its birth almost proclaimed itself a change of paradigm if one only considers the title of the founding article by Guyatt [3]: *Evidence-based medicine. A new approach to teaching the practice of medicine*.

According to Feinstein and Horwitz [20], the true change of paradigm is not situated in the idea of basing the practice of medicine on the integration of the clinical expertise of the practitioner and "the best evidence possible", since it seems to them that medicine has in fact always been practiced this way: the primary change consisted in the primacy given to randomized clinical trials and meta-analyses, which represent the "gold standard". In fact, in two studies published in the early years of Evidence-Based Medicine, it was noted that of 109 hospitalized patients, certainly 82 % of therapeutic decisions were justified by "evidence", but in only 53 % of cases the "evidence" came from a randomized clinical trial, since 29 % of treatments were justified by "convincing non-experimental evidence" [21]. Data of the same type was then published on patients followed in general practice, even inversing the relative importance of randomized trials: 30 % of decisions were based on randomized trials, and 50 % were based on "convincing non-experimental evidence" [22]. This suggests that one of the pillars of Evidence-Based Medicine, the supremacy of the randomized clinical trial, may not correspond to the usual mode of physician decision making, which we will discuss in detail in the rest of this book.

The true change is situated therefore undoubtedly elsewhere. As noted by Kulkarni [23], before the era of Evidence-Based Medicine, the traditional process which moved medicine forward essentially consisted of extrapolation, based on several finite observations of particular cases, of a general conception. This was typically an inductive logic: the more one found similar observations, the greater therefore was the clinical experience, the more one had confidence in the fact that what one had observed would repeat itself similarly in the following case. This is undoubtedly why, in the era before the advent of Evidence-Based Medicine, the publication of retrospective case series of patients was so successful.

On the contrary, Evidence-Based Medicine assumes that there exists at first an objective reality which one can know and which is based on a statistical probability. The method used to study this reality must therefore be based on systematic unbiased observations, whose type example is the randomized clinical trial. Here, the unit of observation is no longer the patient, but instead groups of patients, leading to the concept of *"average patient"*, and the first stage in all randomized clinical trials (in general shown on Table 1 of the publication) is to manage to establish two groups of "average patients" which are identical with regards to the variable that the intervention to be assessed will impact. Here in fact, one does not make observations to arrive at a theory (inductive method): in the case of Evidence-Based Medicine, one tests a hypothesis, which resembles more a hypothetico-deductive method; one begins by the formulation of a null hypothesis which, if it is true, should lead to certain expected observations; if these observations do not occur, one should conclude, with a certain degree of probability, that the null hypothesis is rejected (Kulkarni recognizes nevertheless that this interpretation is subject to caution, since the tested hypothesis itself is based on preliminary observations, and is therefore itself based on inductive logic).

Nevertheless, to be able to approach the objective reality, that is to say to be capable of generating data on which one can base a rational medicine, the process of Evidence-Based Medicine was forced to take another turn, that which consists of decreasing greatly the importance of physiopathological reasoning, preferring only Evidence observed in empirical research (clinical trials): the Evidence, only the Evidence regardless of, in the end, the mechanism. This new disdain for physiopathology has in fact received the support of numerous situations in which hopes had been put in therapeutic strategies developed based on a physiopathological rationale, hopes which were totally let down when these strategies were subjected to the gold standard of the randomized clinical trial: the most famous example is that of deaths in the intervention arm of the trial assessing the effects of antiarrhythmic agents in postinfarction ventricular tachycardia prevention [24].

This is perhaps in fact a true turning point. While the purpose of medical science was in the past to answer questions by decreasing our level of uncertainty particularly through the development of an essentially physiopathological vision of health and diseases, it seems that Evidence-Based Medicine has contributed to questioning the value of this process inherited from Claude Bernard and Pasteur. In medicine, there is no longer "one mechanism, one solution", "one germ, one disease". There are complex situations in which the variability of living things creates an inevitable dimension of uncertainty: Evidence-Based Medicine takes into account this dimension, quantifies it, and integrates it in a method that then becomes capable of helping the practitioner to make her decisions.

## Schrödinger's Cat and Einstein's Boxes

Perhaps this school of thought, integrating the notion of uncertainty, is parallel to that which made physics develop at the start of the twentieth century, of which the Heisenberg uncertainty principle is the emblematic illustration [25]. The fact that uncertainty regarding the result of a bioclinical experiment remains up until its conclusion also brings to mind the paradox of Schrödinger's cat. In 1935, the physicist Erwin Schrödinger imagined an experiment in which he put his cat in a box containing a system which kills the animal as soon as it detects the disintegration of an atom from a radioactive substance present in the box: a Geiger counter is connected to a switch, which causes a hammer to drop breaking a vial containing hydrogen cyanide, which then vaporizes and kills the cat. Let's suppose that the disintegration of the radioactive substance placed in the box has a one in two chance of taking place after 1 min; according to the theory of quantum mechanics, as long as the observation is not made, the atom is *simultaneously* in two states (intact/disintegrated). In the ingenious system imagined by Schrödinger, the cat, in the box, is therefore *both* living and dead, and it is in fact the opening of the box (the observation) which triggers the *choice* between the two states.

Einstein, in a letter to Schrödinger, clarified the paradox by using the following metaphor: if a person places a ball, based on a coin toss, into one of two boxes that she has in front of her, one may certainly say, before opening the box on the left, that there is a one out of two chance that that box will contain the ball; it is a statistical description of the box on the left. However, another description of the box on the left is that there are two distinct possible worlds created by the coin toss: a world where the box on the left contains the ball, and another world, where the box is empty. The only way of deciding between the two worlds is to open the box.

Likewise, in the situation of uncertainty which characterizes therapeutic choice for an individual patient, it is observation of the outcome which will allow one to say if the choice was justified. If it is a matter of mortality, the answer may be received in the very distant future, and may in a number of cases not be available: the doctor may never have the opportunity of opening Einstein's boxes. A qualitative study [26] pointed out the tension general practitioners feel about predicting the clinical course for any one person: "You don't know, do you? You just don't know."

Teaching physicians to reason in this context of uncertainty, is the goal of the endeavor which we have described in this chapter, and, in fact, Evidence-Based Medicine was first presented as an educational method ("a new way to teach medicine"), the purpose being to limit the variability of medical practices. Yet it seems that it undoubtedly encounters obstacles: we have seen in the first part of this book that this objective was far from being reached, perhaps only in half of cases. Might there not be in fact an incompatibility between the principles of the method on which it is based and its applicability by those who are supposed to use it?

## A Critique of Evidence-Based Medicine

We will tackle this critique in three parts: first, we will describe physicians' reactions to the advent of this "new way" to practice medicine; next, we will describe the methodological critiques which were put forth regarding Evidence-Based Medicine; finally, we will present an epistemological critique of its significance.

## The Physician Faced with a New Medicine

Several qualitative studies have aimed to specify physicians' attitudes regarding clinical practice guidelines. In France, Bachimont et al. showed regarding treatment of type 2 diabetes in a survey of 75 physicians having answered a questionnaire that their awareness of the guideline was good, that in general they approved of the content, but that they found that it is too rigid, too distant from clinical reality; general practitioners, they state, often do not have the necessary training, especially regarding lifestyle changes. Finally, certain physicians expressed difficulty announcing a bad result and the lack of a medication that will fix everything: "each time the person is called into question regarding her physical integrity, each time she is expecting a result which will announce that her eyes are beginning to degenerate, something one does not wish to hear, or as late as possible [...] People dream of one thing, having a treatment and we are there to remind them that no" [27, 28]. The overly rigid nature of guidelines, the fact that their implementation takes too much time, even that physicians do not like having activities imposed on them, were also found in a study carried out in 2000 in the Netherlands [29]. Moreover, generalists can have the feeling that guidelines were essentially written by specialists and that they are not directly applicable in their primary care context [26, 30]. The role of lack of time is particularly emphasized [31].

A meta-synthesis, accompanied by a literature review in this field, devoted to physicians' attitudes regarding guidelines, made it possible in fact to distinguish two types of guidelines [32]: those which are essentially prescriptive, recommending to do something (you will...), and those which are proscriptive, recommending to not do something (you will not...). Yet the barriers are not the same: in the first, physicians highlight more the difficulty of applicability of the guideline; in the second, they highlight patients' preferences and the physician-patient relationship which can be obstructed by a guideline which could appear in the eyes of the patient as a rationing of care.

More recently, the study by Lugtenberg et al., of 703 Dutch general practitioners of which 38 % had answered a questionnaire, showed that physicians considered guidelines and their ability to improve the quality of care favorably. The barriers to application most often cited were patients' preferences and lack of applicability of the guideline [33]. The same type of answer was obtained with a questionnaire given to Belgian insurance physicians: this second study, published in 2009, has the value of having asked practitioners their opinion on Evidence-Based Medicine in general. In fact their theoretical knowledge was rather poor, only 56 % of physicians questioned had read up on the question, 50 % had had specific training on Evidence-Based Medicine, and 18 % had become well versed in this approach during their medical studies [34].

Thus, physician compliance with the "new way" to practice medicine appears to be at least mixed. In fact, there appears to be a discrepancy between what Evidence-Based Medicine has the goal of being and what physicians seem to perceive of it: one notes that their critiques focus essentially on guidelines, which represent only the last stage of the process represented in Fig. 5.1, page 48. Yet as we will see, as a whole the process is far from being exempt from critique.

## Theoretical Critiques of Evidence-Based Medicine

Shortly after the publication of the article by the founders of Evidence-Based Medicine, specifying what it is and what it is not [4], critiques, at times severe, were published, leading to detailed responses on the part of the founders or proponents of the method. The first critique was undoubtedly that by Feinstein and Horwitz [20] and one can cite the responses by Straus and McAlister [35] and by Straus and Sackett [36], as well as a vigorous defense of Evidence-Based Medicine by Parker [37].

### Critique of the Supremacy of Randomized Clinical Trials

One should first ask oneself if these are actually safe from bias, which would make them lose the value which they incontestably gain from the fact that they are "randomized". Within the framework of a phenomenological description of clinical inertia, which is the subject of this book, this first critique is significant since in fact one speaks of clinical inertia *in relation* to guidelines. Yet these essentially find their strength in the rigor of randomized clinical trials (or meta-analyses, but the problem is the same since the latter represent in a way an analysis of randomized clinical trials and can therefore suffer from the same critiques).

In fact, Feinstein and Horwitz state [20], randomized clinical trials present major problems: among these, the most significant is that one usually compares two groups of patients, which are in general remarkably "matched" for age, sex, length of the disease, weight, height, initial blood pressure etc., which makes it that on average, the effects of the intervention which one wishes to test will be compared in two groups of "average patients" identical *regarding these parameters*. But what of more subtle or vaguer data, such as the type of symptoms, the progression of the disease, the presence and the severity of comorbidities, tolerance to the treatment if it has already been tried, the psychological profile of the patient, difficulty with adherence, the wishes of the patient, *in short all that the physician in general considers before pronouncing a diagnosis or starting a treatment*? All this data is in general not specified in randomized clinical trials (in any case, they are not presented on "Table I" of the study) – and this is, what's more, clearly why proponents of Evidence-Based Medicine insist upon the fact that its practice does not dispense the physician from taking this into consideration before making her decision: for them, it would therefore be a matter of a fake process [35, 36].

Another critique can also concern one of the methodological aspects of randomized clinical trials whose goal is to reinforce their scientific value, the "intention to treat" analysis of data: at the end of the study, one assess what occurred within each of the two groups, such as they were defined at the time of "randomization", without taking into account what occurred after this time – for example the fact that the patient, in the end took the active medication, even though she was meant to take the placebo, or else that she took it incorrectly due to poor adherence. Of course, this could subsequently, when the medication is taken "in real life", minimize the effects of poor adherence, but does this not cast a doubt on the data regarding, for example, adverse effects of the medication tested, since these can lead to poor adherence during the trial? Incidentally, it should be noted that regarding the consequences of clinical inertia which would be encountered "in real life", they cannot be studied in a randomized clinical trial, since, by definition, investigating physicians have, in a clinical trial in which they participate, *the intention to treat*!

## Who Participates in Studies? Inclusion Criteria

Another major limit of randomized clinical trials is situated in patient inclusion and exclusion criteria, which will define the "average patient" on which the study will be based. On the one hand, choice of a very elevated baseline parameter can increase the chance of having a significant effect, if only by an effect of regression towards the mean. On the other hand, if the criteria are too restrictive, this can decrease the generalization of results of the study: the patient that the physician will be faced with will thus have less chance of resembling the "average patient" from the study. For example one can note that elderly patients are often excluded from clinical trials. Moreover, the presence of multiple diseases in a single patient increases the risk of drug interactions [38], which cannot be foreseen in studies, in which, often, the volunteers have but one disease.

A study precisely examined the "generalizability" of guidelines in the field of hypertension, by studying 16 randomized clinical trials: by "generalizability" one means the capacity of data observed in a specific sample to be able to be applied to the target population. It showed that fewer than 60 % among 34,000 hypertensive American patients could have in fact been enrolled in at least one study: most people were not eligible because of the high levels of diastolic blood pressure that were required to be enrolled in the trials, as well as the age limits for inclusion in the trials [39]. Nevertheless, as noted by Summerskill [40], this way of asking the question (would this patient I have in front of me have been included in the clinical trial) is perhaps less appropriate than to ask oneself if the patient is different from the "average patient" on which the study was based.

### The Nature of Knowledge Coming from Clinical Trials

Tonelli recently insisted [41] upon the fundamental difference between on the one hand, the situation that the physician encounters, when she has to treat this patient she is faced with, and, on the other hand randomized clinical trials, whose purpose is, for example, to demonstrate the effectiveness of a treatment, this demonstration being all the more solid since it is based on a more "average" patient, "identical" in the two groups of individuals which will be compared, thus the need for randomization. This difference between clinical trials, on the one side, and what the physician does in her practice, on the other, suggests that the type of knowledge provided by clinical research is certainly informative but insufficient to be able to be used in medical decisions.

### Patients' Preferences Are Absent from Clinical Trials

Apart from this difference, of an epistemic nature, in the nature of knowledge coming from clinical trials and what is used in "real life", there exists a gap of an ethical nature, that between *the Evidence*, coming from clinical studies, and *the values* of patients on whom one is going to try to implement guidelines coming from this evidence. Yet these are completely absent from the clinical trial itself.

Campbell and Murphy have precisely emphasized that the patient will in any case have a say, expressing thus her preferences: *she's the one who decides*, for example regarding hypertension, how low she wants to go given the side effects, *and not the "targets"*, defined in guidelines based on controlled trials on "the average patient", that can do so [42]. The same can be said regarding diabetes treatment and the risk of hypoglycemia. Here it is a matter of recognizing the role of *the clinical expertise* of patients. Again, this need to integrate patients' preferences, that is to say their values, is clearly indicated as an indispensable complement to all practice of Evidence-Based Medicine [35, 36].

### The Dangers of What Would Be "A New Paradigm"

Replacing one dogmatic medicine by another dogma: Kamhi evokes another risk of Evidence-Based Medicine [13], or at least, of a poor use which risks being made [43], leading one to believe that one can limit the variability of medical practice by developing guidelines, because in fact there would exist one unequivocal solution to one clinical problem, that which is supported by the best *evidence*: "By presuming that there is one best course of action, Evidence-Based Medicine has the potential to create the kind of dogmatic certainty that it was designed to eliminate."

But especially, to see in the emergence of Evidence-Based Medicine a true "new paradigm", rather than a process which helps physicians to work in the context of uncertainty which is theirs, would present major dangers: the risk of a diversion of research policies, consisting of promoting themes capable of leading to guidelines and, thus, to the benefit of the pharmaceutical industry, therefore orienting scientific research towards medications for common diseases more than towards interventions on lifestyle or orphan diseases [37]: in fact, research regarding the latter is in both cases more difficult to implement, and their results would be undoubtedly less profitable in terms of financial repercussions.

One could also fear that a dogmatic vision of Evidence-Based Medicine as a so called "new paradigm", in light of which everything can be scientifically evaluated, influences profoundly the health care system in general, leading also to ranking of therapeutic strategies and deciding on Manichaean foundations (it's "proven" or it's not) the reimbursement of medication, support for development of non-drug therapeutic strategies etc. It could lead in fact to a rationing of care.

## Guidelines That Are Numerous, Long, at Times Contradictory or Questionable

Among their critiques of Evidence-Based Medicine, Feinstein and Horwitz [20] cited the risk that physicians pass less time at the patient's bedside, being busier at the library or in front of their computer. In fact, as of 1998, one publication showed that the primary barrier to implementation of the principles of Evidence-Based Medicine by general practitioners was lack of time [44]. Guidelines are more and more numerous and longer and longer. Of course there exist summaries, but the physician who, almost inevitably, is forced to make do with reading them, risks missing the subtleties which are found in the full version [42]. Bobrie et al. also noted, in the field of hypertension as elsewhere, the multiplication of guidelines [45]. Moreover they insist upon the fact that guidelines in a given field are often different, both in the patient populations to which they apply, but also in what is recommended [46]. The problem of the length of guidelines was also brought up by Stone et al. [47] and by the study by Kang et al., carried out in the field of asthma on Korean physicians, showing their preference for advice on asthma medications, gradation of the severity of the disease, decision trees, and practical presentation in the form of laminated cards or electronic documents [48].

Perhaps guidelines would benefit from being written in simple and, especially, specific terms. One can show, based on behavioral considerations that the fact that a guideline is specific decreases the feeling of uncertainty which leads to inaction: for example it may be important that the guideline clearly presents answers to the questions "who, what, where, when, how" to implement the guideline [49].

Finally, the fact that guidelines change with new *evidence*, but also that some among them can be challenged for procedural reasons (for example when it appears simply that the experts that developed them did not clearly disclose their conflicts of interest), does not incite physicians to comply, in general, with the principles of Evidence-Based Medicine.

## Epistemological Critique of the Concept of Evidence-Based Medicine

In his book *The Reflective Practitioner, How Professionals Think in Action* [50], Donald Schön described the crisis of confidence in the value of professional knowledge which "*practitioners*" (this term is used in a generic and not only medical way) encountered in the middle of the last century. This crisis, he says, is linked to the divergence which has emerged between the "knowledge" used by a given profession and five new conditions of professional practice, marked by complexity, uncertainty, instability, uniqueness, and value conflict.

This applies perfectly to the medical context: (1) *complexity*; for example, physicians must devise their actions within a health care system which they do not understand and do not control; (2) *uncertainty*; all that we have described previously bears witness: as Schön states more generally, "problems are interconnected, environments are turbulent, and the future is indeterminate"; (3) *instability*; the role of physicians is molded constantly by medical progress and the reorganization of the health care system: "the patterns of task and knowledge are inherently unstable"; (4) *uniqueness*; Schön cites what one of his physician friends told him: "85 percent of the problems a doctor sees in his office are not in the book"; (5) finally, *value conflict*; for example, one must recognize the fact that physicians could feel torn between the imperative of the quality of care and bureaucratic pressure to increase efficiency.

Schön shows in his book that there is a crisis, because, faced with this new practical reality, traditional professional expertise continues to be based on the paradigm of a Technical Rationality, proposing that the knowledge which a "practitioner" uses can be described on three levels: basic sciences, applied sciences, and the skills to use this basic and applied science (the distinction between basic and clinical sciences is familiar to all those having completed their medical studies). For Schön, this paradigm of the Technical Rationality of the "practitioner" comes directly from Positivism, stipulating that all questions can be resolved scientifically, including questions relating to practice: "Given agreement on ends, the question 'How ought I to act?' could be reduced to a merely instrumental question about the means best suited to achieve one's ends." The key is therefore to clearly formulate the question, since the problem could then be resolved by a process coming from a calculation of probabilities.

Can Technical Rationality help the "practitioner" to resolve a practical problem? In fact, the difficulty that she encounters is not here. It is not a matter of *resolving* a problem, but rather of *formulating* it, within the context of the five current conditions of practice, described above: as Schön states, "In real-world practice, problems do not present themselves to the practitioner as givens. They must be constructed from the materials of problematic situations which are puzzling, troubling, and uncertain. In order to convert a problematic situation to a problem, a practitioner must do a certain kind of work. He must make sense of an uncertain situation that initially makes no sense." Yet, Schön states, formulation of the problem is an indispensable stage to being able to resolve it, *but it could itself not fall within Technical Rationality.* If one comes back to Evidence-Based Medicine, we have seen that its practice faced with a given patient begins with a stage of formulation of the question, according to the PICO method. Of course, this increases the chance of finding an answer, but this "translation" can lead to an answer which does not correspond to the initial question. In fact it often occurs that certain questions remain unanswered, or else that the answers given are not clear [51].

For Schön, and it is the primary message of his book, formulation of the problem by the practitioner falls under, not Technical Rationality, but rather what he calls Reflection-in-Action: this is that know-how which the practitioner is not always able to describe and which is based on the inventive improvisation learned in practice.

Schön published his book in 1983, therefore well before the term Evidence-Based Medicine was forged. Yet, if we come back to the latter, *it appears in fact to typically fall within the paradigm of "Technical Rationality"*: this epistemological critique implies that Evidence-Based Medicine may not be able to resolve the difficulties which physicians currently encounter in their practice, this discrepancy explaining therefore, at least in part, the occurrence of what one calls clinical inertia.

## From an Evidence-Based Medicine to a Practice-Based Medicine

One understands therefore that, in the reasoning which leads her to make a clinical decision, the physician does not, in any case, use only the data from Evidence-Based Medicine. We have already cited studies suggesting that it is undoubtedly used in only one quarter of medical decisions.

Tonelli emphasized the supremacy given to the "Evidence" by Evidence-Based Medicine, compared to data from physician clinical expertise and physiopathological reasoning, which, it's been shown, were somewhat scorned by Evidence-Based Medicine [41]. In fact, according to him, the physician calls upon five foundations to make a clinical decision: (1) of course, the results of clinical research and what she knows of evidence-based medicine, but also (2) her clinical experience, (3) physiopathological reasoning, (4) patients' preferences, and (5) her environment.

Yet, Tonelli states, the knowledge provided by the first three elements is, from an epistemic point of view, of a different nature *and cannot be hierarchized*. Based on this premise, this author proposes a Case-Based Approach, consisting first, for the physician, to ask herself if the patient in front of her resembles sufficiently the "average patient" so that she can apply the data from Evidence-Based Medicine on her; if this is not the case, the physician must ask if the patient resembles patients from her own clinical experience, possibly calling upon the experience of her colleagues; she should not hesitate to use physiopathological data; finally she must integrate patients' preferences in her decision. Thus, other approaches aiming to provide evidence are beginning to emerge, combining with the methodology of Evidence-Based Medicine the data of Practice-Based Evidence [52].

Parker [37] suggests, in order to not end up throwing the Randomized Clinical Trial baby out with the bathwater, to admit that, *statistically*, it remains the methodology having the highest level of evidence, but that there are situations where other types of high level evidence can be considered, and that all prioritization in this field must take into account individually the different medical issues. This flexibility could be welcome. Evidence-Based Medicine is therefore no longer a rigid endeavor which at the same time threatens the freedom of the physician by producing restrictive guidelines and represents a prompt to paternalistic behavior which, in return, would limit the freedom of the patient: it is the very condition of clinical freedom; in these conditions, the proponents and the critics of Evidence-Based Medicine can come together on the idea that medicine is both an art and a science [37].

But once the collected data, the Evidence, is used to lead to the development of best *practices*, that is to say once one passes from knowledge to action, given that knowledge, as demonstrated in this chapter is necessarily marred with uncertainty, it is essential that this be clearly mentioned in the guideline [53].

## By Way of Provisional Conclusion: Guidelines or "Mindlines"?

In summary, it appears that Evidence-Based Medicine represents a rational endeavor, involving both the physician and the patient, aiming to give the physician in a context of uncertainty the possibility to offer her patient the best treatment available, based on the best scientific data. This allows one to specify in particular the qualities of diagnostic tests involved and the chances of success of proposed treatments. Based on this Evidence, it makes possible the development of guidelines which would help the practitioner to make the best choice, all while reminding her on the one hand that she must always ask herself if the guideline applies to the patient she is faced with, and on the other hand that she must take into account the preferences of this patient. The purpose of these guidelines is clearly to lead to a standardization of practices, so that all patients can benefit from better care.

With a didactic intention, application of Bayes' theorem can be simplified by giving it a qualitative form [54]. This shows clearly that implementation of Evidence-Based Medicine is not at all intuitive. In fact, even if physicians know and approve of the principles of Evidence-Based Medicine and guidelines, one can ask if it is not illusionary to imagine that they use concretely and comfortably its "process" in stages, such as it has been described at the beginning of this chapter, when they have to, on a day-to-day basis, make a decision for the patient they have in front of them: formulation of the question, search for the best "evidence", critique of this evidence, application to the patient etc. [55, 56]. On the contrary, when Schön speaks of Reflection-in-Action [50], he evokes this capacity of the "practitioner" to act, consisting of the use of implicit rules which it would be very difficult for her to describe, that she has formed herself through a reflection conducted constantly during her practice: in summary, this "art" which makes her an expert able to act in a context of complexity, instability, uncertainty, uniqueness and value conflict.

In a more analytical way, Gabbay and le May [57] therefore proposed, in an ethnographic type approach, that physicians on a day-to-day basis do not use "guidelines", but instead "mindlines", that is to say mental combinations of information developed based on different sources: certainly the guidelines themselves, but also what they learned during their studies and their training, their own clinical experience, discussions they have with their local colleagues or those they encounter during post-graduate training sessions or conventions, their interactions with patients, finally what "opinion leaders" tell them; incidentally, the latter have an important responsibility since they will "guide the opinion", and it is important that they themselves, at least, base the messages that they disseminate on Evidence alone.

The influence, in the production of these "mindlines", of the information that physicians (including "opinion leaders") receive from the pharmaceutical industry during medical visits, conventions sponsored by the above or all other types of interactions, should not be underestimated [58–62]. This information can be biased for commercial purposes. One must also keep in mind that a great number of large studies on which Evidence-Based Medicine is based were "sponsored" by the pharmaceutical industry, from the conception of the study to the analysis of the results, even to the writing of the article, then to its public presentation by "opinion leaders". This is the importance on the one hand of the regulatory aspects which must frame the medical visit, and on the other hand of the critical thinking which the physician (including the "opinion leader"!) must be able to demonstrate regarding this information, the teaching of which should be part of all medical training; this is also the urgent need to rigorously eliminate the possible impact of "conflicts of interest" during the development of guidelines, which has just been reinforced by the French legislative apparatus, especially following the Mediator affair [63].

The desire to arrive at a standardization of practices [64] – or at a decrease in their variability – was at the origin, as has been shown historically speaking, of the development of Evidence-Based Medicine. One can ask if one should not revisit this position and if, on the contrary, the future might not go towards an individualization of therapeutic processes, with for example the development of pharmacogenetics. Even while waiting for these developments, Evidence-Based Medicine has stated time and again that guidelines must take into account the individual patient; the physician also knows that an "à la carte" treatment is often preferable over the application of a generic guideline, particularly in the case of patients with multiple diseases or polypharmacy, that is to say which might not resemble the "average patient" which was included in the large clinical trial which led to the development of the guideline. The difficulty is therefore to make the patient enter into a category which benefits from a specific treatment. Veazie et al. proposed that clinical inertia could result from this difficulty, for physicians, to appropriately "categorize" patients [65]. This could explain why clinical inertia is more frequent, we have seen, in elderly patients who often have several diseases and are treated with numerous medications. Incidentally, in the field of diabetes care, the recent consensus proposed jointly by the American Diabetes Association [66] and the European

Association for the Study of Diabetes Mellitus [67] is based on an individualization of guidelines, concerning both the definition of the target (glycated hemoglobin) and the choice of the medication. This individualized guideline helps physicians in "categorizing" patients. It may decrease clinical inertia [68].

In fact, many postulates behind Evidence-Based Medicine, not only are not intuitive for the physician and for the patient, but, as we will see, can even be counterintuitive. For example, regarding patients, when one says that good practice of Evidence-Based Medicine must take into account their preferences, the "utility" they see in what is proposed to them, can one not expect that, for their part, they could experience difficulty in specifying their preferences in a quantified way, for example deciding that if death has a "utility" equal to zero, and being cured equal to 1, living with the consequences of an amputation or hemiplegia has a "utility" of 0.3? [69] The decision, for the patient, of a "*preference*" is perhaps not as obvious as the rationality of Evidence-Based Medicine would well like to imagine.

Thus, evoking the complexity of determinants that mentally guide the physician in her practice, her "mindlines" [57], which make it that she is, as Schön stated, a "reflective practitioner" [50], allows one perhaps to explain why compliance to an "official" guideline, is always but one of the elements which intervenes in medical decisions. Therefore, one can no longer be surprised to observe that sometimes physicians do not follow official clinical practice guidelines: in certain cases at least, these are in fact "reflective practitioners"; their inaction is appropriate, and, as noted by Serge Halimi and Claude Attali, who refer to Schön's book, this inaction is what's more in fact an action [70]. In our previous work devoted to patient therapeutic adherence [71], we have likewise shown that the fact that patients, for example, do *not* take a pill, could also represent an *action*, that is to say an event caused by a reason [72].

*

* *

In fact, as we will see, physicians, in the shaping of their reasons to act, are what's more subjected to many cognitive biases that jeopardize the very rationality of the intellectual endeavor, which one could refer to as "Bayesian", which aims to establish Evidence-Based Medicine: in the following chapter, we will see in fact that physicians can act neither in compliance with guidelines that the latter proposes and which they appear to know and even approve, nor even, *in fact, with their own "mindlines", with their own reasons*.

It's here that clinical inertia puzzles us the most, when it appears as a failure to take action - a failure to act, stated Phillips – which is in contradiction with what the physician knows she should do: this apparently irrational nature of clinical inertia requires one to attempt a more in-depth critique of what we will call *medical reason*.

## References

1. Goodman KW. Ethics and Evidence-Based Medicine. Cambridge: Cambridge University Press; 2003. p. 5–6.
2. Cochrane AL. 1931–1971: a critical review, with particular reference to the medical profession. In: Medicines for the year 2000. London: Office of Health Economics; 1979. p. 1–11.

# References

3. Evidence Based Medicine Working Group. Evidence-Based Medicine. A new approach to teaching the practice of medicine. JAMA. 1992;268:2420–5.
4. Sackett DL, Rosenberg WMC, Gray JAM, Haynes RB, Richardson WS. Evidence based medicine: what it is and what it isn't. BMJ. 1996;312:71–2.
5. Delvenne C, Pasleau F. Comment résoudre en pratique un problème diagnostique ou thérapeutique en suivant une démarche EBM? Rev Med Liege. 2000;55:226–32.
6. Smith GCS, Pell JC. Parachute use to prevent death and major trauma related to gravitational challenge: systematic review of randomised controlled trials. BMJ. 2003;327. doi:10.1136/bmj.327.7429.1459.
7. Haute Autorité de Santé: Élaboration de Recommandations de Bonne Pratique. Méthode. "Recommandations pour la pratique clinique". 2010. Annexe 3, p. 19.
8. Haynes B, Haines A. Getting research findings into practice. Barriers and bridges to evidence based clinical practice. BMJ. 1998;317:273–6.
9. Haynes RB. Loose connections between peer-reviewed clinical journals and clinical practice. Ann Intern Med. 1990;113:724–8.
10. Cochrane Reviews. The Cochrane Collaboration. http://www2.cochrane.org/reviews/. Accessed 20 Apr 2014.
11. Westerneck TB, Pak MH. Using clinical practice guidelines to improve patient care. Wis Med J. 2005;104:30–3.
12. Straus SE, Richardson WS, Glasziou P, Haynes RB. Evidence-Based Medicine: how to teach and practice EBM. Elsevier; 2005. p. 208.
13. Kamhi AG. Balancing certainty and uncertainty in clinical practice. Lang Speech Hear Serv Sch. 2011;42:59–64.
14. Bayes T, Price M. An essay towards solving a problem in the doctrine of chances. Philos Trans R Soc Lond. 1763;53:370–418.
15. Mayer D. Essential Evidence-Based Medicine. New York: Cambridge University Press; 2004. p. 249.
16. Straus SE, Richardson WS, Glasziou P, Haynes RB. Evidence-Based Medicine: how to teach and practice EBM. Elsevier; 2005. p. 156.
17. Sox HC, Blatt MA, Higgins MC, Marton KI. Medical decision making. Philadelphia: American College of Physicians; 2007. p. 169–200.
18. Kuhn TS. The structure of scientific revolutions. Chicago: University of Chicago Press; 1962.
19. Howick J. The philosophy of Evidence-Based Medicine. Oxford: Wiley-Blackwell; 2011. p. 10.
20. Feinstein AR, Horwitz RL. Problems in the "evidence" of "Evidence-based Medicine". Am J Med. 1997;103:529–35.
21. Ellis J, Mulligan I, Rowe J, Sackett DL. Inpatient general medicine is evidence based. Lancet. 1995;346:407–9.
22. Gill P, Dowell AC, Neal RD, Smith N, Heywood P, Wilson AE. Evidence based general practice: a retrospective study of interventions in one training practice. BMJ. 1996;312:8819–21.
23. Kulkarni A. The challenges of Evidence-Based Medicine: a philosophical perspective. Med Health Care Philos. 2005;8:255–60.
24. The Cardiac Arrhytmia Suppression Trial (CAST) Investigators. Preliminary Report: effect of encainamide and flecainide on mortality in a randomized trial of arrhytmia suppression after myocardial infarction. N Engl J Med. 1989;321:406–12.
25. Bursztajn AJ, Feinbloom RI, Hamon RM, Brodsky A. Medical choices, medical chances: how patients, families and physicians can cope with uncertainty. New York: iUniverse; 1990.
26. Freeman AC, Sweeney K. Why general practitioners do not implement evidence: qualitative study. BMJ. 2001;323:1100–2.
27. Bachimont J, Cogneau J, Letourmy A. Pourquoi les médecins généralistes n'observent-ils pas les recommandations de bonnes pratiques cliniques ? L'exemple du diabète de type 2. Sciences Sociales et Santé. 2006;24:75–103.
28. Cogneau J, Lehr-Drylewicz AM, Bachimont J, Letourmy A. Ecarts entre le référentiel et la pratique dans le diabète de type 2. Les préjugés des médecins et des patients sont un obstacle à une éducation efficace des patients. Presse Med. 2007;36:764–70.
29. Dijkstra R, Braspenning J, Uiters E, van Ballegooie E, Grol RT. Perceived barriers to the implementation of diabetes guidelines in hospitals in the Netherlands. Neth J Med. 2000; 56:80–5.

30. Price D, Thomas M. Breaking new ground: challenging existing asthma guidelines. BMC Pulm Med. 2006;6 Suppl 1:S6. doi:10.1186/1471-2466-6-S1-S6.
31. Hobbs FD, Erhardt L. Acceptance of guideline recommendations and perceived implementation of coronary heart disease prevention among primary care physicians in five European countries: the Reassessing European Attitudes about Cardiovascular Treatment (REACT) survey. Fam Pract. 2002;19:596–604.
32. Carlsen B, Glenton C, Pope C. Thou shalt versu thou shalt not: a meta-synthesis of GPs' attitudes to clinical practice guidelines. Br J Gen Pract. 2007;57:971–8.
33. Lugtenberg M, Burgers JS, Besters CF, Han D, Westert GP. Perceived barriers to guideline adherence: a survey among general practitioners. BMC Fam Pract. 2011;12:98.
34. Heselmans A, Donceel P, Aertgeerts B, Van de Velde S, Ramaekers D. The attitude of begian social insurance physicians towards evidence-based practice and clinical practice guidelines. BMC Fam Pract. 2009;10:64. doi:10.1186/1471-2296-10-64.
35. Straus SE, McAlister FA. Evidence-vased medicine: a commentary on common criticisms. CMAJ. 2000;163:837–41.
36. Straus SE, Sackett DL. Applying evidence to the individual patient. Ann Oncol. 1999;10: 29–32.
37. Parker M. False dichotomies: EBM, clinical freedom, and the art of medicine. J Med Ethics Med Humanit. 2005;31:23–30.
38. Tinetti ME, Bogardus ST, Agostini JV. Potential pitfalls of disease-specific guidelines for patients with multiple conditions. N Engl J Med. 2004;351:2870–4.
39. Pedone C, Lapane KL. Generalizability of guidelines and physicians' adherence. Case study on the Sixth Joint National Committe's guidelines on hypertension. BMC Public Health. 2003;3:24. doi:10.1186/1471-2458-3-24.
40. Summerskill W. Evidence-based practice and the individual. Lancet. 2005;365:13–4.
41. Tonelli MR. Integrating clinical research into clinical decision making. Ann Ist Super Sanita. 2011;47:26–30.
42. Campbell NC, Murchie P. Treating hypertension with guidelines in general practice. Patients decide how low they go, no targets. BMJ. 2004;329:523–4.
43. Justice L. Evidence-based terminology. Am J Speech Lang Pathol. 2008;17:324–5.
44. McColl A, Smith H, White P, Field J. General practitioners' perceptions of the route to evidence based medicine: a questionnaire survey. BMJ. 1998;316:361–5.
45. Bobrie G, Durieux P, Postel-Vinay N, Plouin PF. De l'observation clinique à l'évaluation des pratiques: les recommandations pour la prise en charge de l'hypertension artérielle. Néphrologie et Thérapeutique. 2009;5:S240–5.
46. Georg G, Colombet I, Durieux P, Ménard J, Meneton P. A comparative analysis of four clinical guidelines for hypertension management. J Hum Hypertens. 2008;22:829–37.
47. Stone TT, Schweikart SB, Mantese A, Sonnad SS. Guideline attribute and implementation preferences among physicians in multiple health systems. Qual Manag Health Care. 2005;14:177–87.
48. Kang MK, Kim BK, Kim TW, Kang HR, Park HW, Chang YS, Kim SS, Min KU, Kim YY, Cho SH. Physicians' preferences for asthma guidelines implementation. Allergy Asthm Immunol Res. 2010;2:247–53.
49. Michie S, Johnston M. Changing clinical behaviour by making guidelines specific. BMJ. 2004;328:343–5.
50. Schön DA. The reflective practitioner. How professionals think in action. New York: Basic Books; 1983.
51. Ely JW, Osheroff JA, Maviglia SM, Rosenbaum MME. Patient-care questions that physicians are unable to answer. J Am Med Inform Assoc. 2007;14:1407–14.
52. Horn SD, Gassaway J, Pentz L, James R. Practice-based evidence for clinical practice improvement: an alternative study design for Evidence-Based Medicine. In: Hovenga EJS et al., editors. Health informatics. IOS Press; 2010. p. 446–60.
53. Woolf SH. Do clinical practice guidelines define good medical care? The need for good science and the disclosure of uncertainty when defining best practices. Chest. 1998;113:166S–71.

# References

54. Medow MA, Lucey CR. A qualitative approach to Bayes' theorem. Evid Based Med. 2011. doi:10.1136/ebm-2011-0007.
55. Lewis JP, Tully MP. The discomfort of an evidence-based prescribing decision. J Eval Clin Pract. 2009;15:1152–8.
56. Reid MC, Lane DA, Feinstein AR. Academic calculations versus clinical judgments: practicing physicians' use of quantitative measures of test accuracy. Am J Med. 1998;104:374–80.
57. Gabbay J, le May A. Evidence based guidelines or collectively constructed "mindlines"? Ethnographic study of knowledge management in primary care. BMJ. 2004;329:1013–7.
58. Gill PS, Freemantle N, Bero L, Haaijer-Ruskamp F, Markela M, Barjesteh KP. GPs' prescribing behaviour may be affected by drug promotion. BMJ. 1996;313:367.
59. Lexchin J. Interactions between physicians and the pharmaceutical industry: what does the literature say? Can Med Assoc J. 1993;149:1402–22.
60. Armstrong D, Reyburn H, Jones R. A study of general practitioner's reasons for changing their prescribing behaviour. BMJ. 1996;312:949–52.
61. Zipkin DA, Steinman MA. Interactions between pharmaceutical representatives and doctors in training. A thematic review. J Gen Intern Med. 2005;20:777–86.
62. Chen MM, Landefeld CS. Physicians' behavior and their interactions with drug companies. JAMA. 1994;271:684–9.
63. Loi n°2011–2012 du 29 Décembre 2011 relative au renforcement de la sécurité sanitaire du médicament et des produits de santé, JORF n° 0302 du 30 décembre 2011. p. 22667.
64. Morris AH. The importance of protocol-directed patient management for research on lung-protective ventilation. In: Dreyfuss D, Saumon G, Hubamyr R, editors. Ventilator-induced lung injury. New York: Taylor and Francis Group; 2006. p. 537–610.
65. Veazie PJ, Johnson PE, O'Connor PJ. Is there a downside to customizing care? Implications of general and patient-specific treatment strategies. J Eval Clin Pract. 2009;15:1171–6.
66. Inzuchi SE, Bergenstal RM, Buse JB, et al. Management of hyperglycemia in type2 diabetes: a patient-centered approach. Position Statement of the American Diabetes Association (ADA) and the European Association for the Study of Diabetes (EASD). Diabetes Care. 2012;35:1364–79.
67. Inzuchi SE, Bergenstal RM, Buse JB, et al. Management of hyperglycemia in type2 diabetes: a patient-centered approach. Position Statement of the American Diabetes Association (ADA) and the European Association for the Study of Diabetes (EASD). Diabetologia. 2012;55:1577–96.
68. Reach G. Clinical inertia, uncertainty and individualized guidelines. Diabetes Metab. 2014. doi:10.1016/j.diabet.2013.12.009.
69. Balla JI, Elstein AS, Christensen C. Obstacles to acceptance of clinical decision analysis. BMJ. 1989;298:579–82.
70. Halimi S, Attali C. L'inertie thérapeutique dans le diabète de type 2: la comprendre sans la banaliser. Médecine des Maladies Métaboliques. 2011;5 Suppl 2:S62–8.
71. Reach G. The mental mechanisms of patient adherence to long term therapies, mind and care, Foreword by Pascal Engel, "Philosophy and Medicine" series, Springer, forthcoming
72. Davidson D. Actions, reasons and causes, Journal of Philosophy, 1963, repris comme Essai 1 de Action et événements, traduction et préface de P. Engel, P.U.F., Collection Épiméthée, 1993.

# To Do or Not to Do: A Critique of Medical Reason

**6**

## Abstract

This central chapter of the book proposes an analysis of the psychology of medical decisions, often based on mental processes called heuristics, described in particular by Kahneman and Tversky and that have the advantage of rapidity: for example the representativeness heuristic has us ask how the patient in front of us resembles patients in a specific category, or the availability heuristic has us assess the probability of an event by the ease with which we can recall having already seen it. We also evoke the importance of loss aversion, described by Kahneman and Tversky in their Prospect Theory. Yet the use of these heuristics presents a risk of bias and error. We also analyze the effect of emotions, in particular the avoidance of regret in medical reasoning, while feelings are absent in Evidence-Based Medicine. We conclude that the discordance between the Technical Rationality of Evidence-Based Medicine, relying on the unbiased methodology of randomized clinical trials and the "medical reason" of the physician, which relies on heuristics and emotions with their risk of bias, represents a general explanation of clinical inertia, which can be seen as a preference for the status quo.

## Definition

We call *medical reason* all mental mechanisms which lead the physician and the patient, for the one, to offer a treatment, and for the other, to be "adherent" and to follow the medical prescription. The goal of this chapter is attempt to describe the complexity of these mechanisms.

In our previous work [1], we proposed a model of patient adherence involving mental states such as knowledge, beliefs, desires, emotions, pain, pleasure etc. (Fig. 6.1). This model is called "intentionalist" because the mental states are for the

© Springer International Publishing Switzerland 2015
G. Reach, *Clinical Inertia: A Critique of Medical Reason*,
DOI 10.1007/978-3-319-09882-1_6

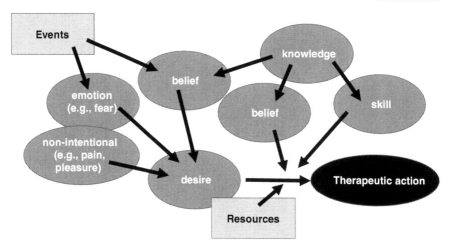

**Fig. 6.1** The *medical reason* of adherence (Extracted from Ref. [1])

most part mental states called "intentional", as defined by philosophers like John Searle [2], that is to say, attitudes having content: in the belief "I believe it is raining", the attitude is a belief, and "it is raining" is the content of the belief. These mental states constitute the "medical reason" of the patient when she must carry out a task for her treatment (therapeutic action).

According to this model, desire, placed at the center of the figure, represents the attitude which leads to action: for example my desire to lose a few pounds causes me to sign up at the gym, as my physician recommended. A belief, associated with desire, essentially plays an instrumental role: here, I am adherent – I carry out the therapeutic action which was prescribed – because I believe that this action is part of those which will have my desire, to lose a few pounds, be fulfilled. The desire can in turn be caused by another belief—for example, I believe that having lost a few pounds, I'll impress my friends, and this causes my desire to lose weight—or by an emotion—I imagine the pride that I'll feel at the thought of having managed to lose the weight. Skills also play an instrumental role in action—I know what I should do, avoid fatty foods and increase my physical activity, but this is not why I do it: before having made the decision to lose weight, I knew this and yet I didn't do it. Finally, my beliefs and my skills, which I have just described, are forged based on what I know: my knowledge of dietetics.

In this model, presented in Fig. 6.1, emotions play a major role in inducing revisions of beliefs and desires [3]. For example, it can be the birth of my grandchildren which triggered my desire to commit to a health behavior. It is evident that non-intentional factors (not having content), such as pain or pleasure can have a motivational role. Moreover, events can also intervene as a *substratum* of new beliefs, or by causing the occurrence of emotions through the difference between the old situation and the new [3]. Exogenous factors, such as the existence of or the lack of resources (disadvantaged) for example, can intervene to encourage or on the contrary limit patient adherence. Finally, according to Searle, different mental states described here are entrenched in an entire Background, of skills and presuppositions, which allow them to "function". Events, mental states and exogenous factors can have a positive or negative effect on patient adherence. For I can also not do all that my "reason" tells me to do, or stop doing it. It should be noted that beliefs intervene on several levels in this model, as does the important role of emotions and resources.

We have proposed that the same model can be used to represent the *medical reason* which intervenes, this time in the mind of the physician, to lead her to make – or not make – a medical prescription [4]. Here, it is a matter of, for example, explaining the physician's compliance – or noncompliance, that is to say the clinical inertia regarding a guideline: the mental states which intervene are her knowledge, what she learned during her studies or during continuing medical education, or else what she has seen while reading a guideline which has just been published; her skills were forged by her experience as a practitioner; she also has beliefs which she is less sure of; she is also prey to her emotions, remembering for example an unfortunate side effect which occurred recently in a patients for which she had followed the guideline in question; obviously, the resources which she has at her disposal intervene also. In the end, what is represented, in the case of the physician, in Fig. 6.1, are the "mindlines" which we have mentioned at the end of the previous chapter [5].

This suggests that the two phenomena of patient nonadherence and physician clinical inertia can be seen as one of the two possible outcomes of the implementation of *medical reason*, the other consequence being on the contrary that the patient follows the medical prescription and that the physician follows the guideline. Even if the first possibility, from a normative point of view, can be considered as unfortunate, one must insist that it would be wrong to describe it as a "failure" of medical reason: as we will see, medical reason is based on mechanisms which bring with them the possibility that the patient be nonadherent and the physician clinically inert.

In order to explain the mechanisms which preside over clinical inertia, we propose indeed to show that it is the consequence of cognitive biases liable to intervene in all human decision making in a context of uncertainty and risk: in particular we will bring to light the role of simplified modes of reasoning, called heuristics, in decision making, and that of emotions, elements that are both integrative and potentially disruptive of what we have called medical reason. Incidentally, the same reflection could be useful for revisiting the mental mechanisms underlying the phenomenon of patient nonadherence [1].

## The Context of Uncertainty Which Surrounds All Medical Activities, and the Concept of Risk

In the previous chapter, we have shown that the variability of biological phenomena introduced uncertainty regarding the results of tests (explaining for example the existence of falsely positive or negative results) and treatments (explaining the impossibility to predict other than by statistical data the results of medical prescriptions, regarding both the effectiveness and the side effects of treatments). In fact, this uncertainty can be seen from another angle if one considers that it concerns a decision: it leads to tackling the concept of risk.

Thus, Kahneman and Tversky make the distinction between a decision without risk (for example accepting a transaction in which a good is exchanged against a certain sum of money) and a decision under risk, in which one accepts a bet which can lead to, with a certain probability, the gain of a certain sum of money [6]. When the physician must decide on a treatment which can have several outcomes, such as they were represented in Fig. 5.4 page 56, she is typically placed in a situation under risk, and we have indicated how a calculation of probabilities can allow her to make a shared decision with the patient, taking into account the preferences of the latter, expressed in the form of respective values – or "utilities" – that the patient gives to different possible outcomes of the proposed treatment, allowing one to calculate for each outcome an "expected utility" by multiplying the value of the utility by the probability of this outcome.

## The Notion of Heuristics and Bias

This calculation of probability, consisting of adding together "expected utilities" is in truth what one expects of an agent in the classic theories of rational choice. Nevertheless as of the middle of the last century, it was realized that individuals, when they have to make decisions in a context of uncertainty, do not usually engage in statistical calculations of this type, due to the limited nature of human intellectual capacities [7].

In fact, particularly through the founding contribution in this field by Amos Tversky (1937–1996) and Daniel Kahneman (born in 1934, Nobel Prize in Economics in 2002) one became aware of the fact that, faced with these complex situations, human beings use intuitive judgment processes, called "heuristics", which are categorically different than those proposed by classic models of rationality. These are "mental short-cuts", reasoning that is much simpler and quicker to implement than complex calculations of probability. In order to explain what a heuristic is, one can give as example the way in which someone tries to answer the question: what is the frequency of cocaine addiction among Hollywood actors? To answer the question, she would try to recall examples of cocaine addicts among the American actors that she knows. Heuristics have the advantage of being easy to implement, but they present the inconvenience of being able to give wrong answers, what one calls a "bias", that is to say the difference between the judgment that one pronounces by using the heuristic and that which one would pronounce by using normative, for example purely statistical, rules.

## Different Heuristics Used in Human Judgment Within a Context of Uncertainty

In their founding article [8], Tversky and Kahneman described several types of heuristics:

1. **Representativeness heuristic**: when one has to answer a question of the type: what is the probability that an object A belongs to class B, or that an event A is caused by a process B, or that a process B can cause an event A (we note that these are the type of questions which are usually posed in the medical field!) one often uses a "representativeness heuristic" which consists of assessing this probability based on the degree to which A is representative of B, that is to say *A resembles B*. The use of a heuristic of this type is what's more largely used in the diagnosis stage. Pat Croskerry gives the following example: if a 40 year old man, up to then in good health, arrives at the hospital emergency room with lower back pain, nausea, vomiting and hematuria, we immediately evoke a diagnosis of renal colic. This mental short-cut saves us from having to evoke one by one all the differential diagnoses which could connect all these symptoms; and, *most often*, we are right [9]. That's the full positive value of heuristics, which we will come back to.

Nevertheless, this heuristic can be a major source of bias: in particular, the fact that A resembles B does not take into account the prevalence of B. If for example, the clinical presentation of patient A resembles that which is most often observed in the case of malaria, but if malaria is in fact very rare in the environment in which one observes patient A, the observed resemblance does not make it more likely that A has malaria. Yet it's been shown that Bayes' theorem begins by assessing the pre-test probability, that is to say the prevalence. In other words, this implies that the use of heuristics can bias the results of Bayesian reasoning.

Another consequence of the representativeness heuristic can be illustrated by the following example: medical students are given a fictional scenario of a patient with clinical evidence suggesting a stroke. Telling them that her breath smells of alcohol decreases their capacity to make this diagnosis: the student has not use Bayes' theorem (what is the pre-test probability that the patient has had a stroke, what is the sensitivity and the specificity of a alcohol breath), but used a representativeness heuristic: patients in group B who smell of alcohol and who are in a coma, often, are under the influence of alcohol, and the fact of smelling of alcohol makes it that *patient A resembles patients in group B*: the student will wrongly pronounce a diagnosis of drunken stupor. Payne showed that it occurs often that one uses this representativeness heuristic, forgetting the importance of the prevalence of diseases, preferring reasoning of a causal nature [10].

Conversely, a study showed that physicians, faced with patients of a different culture or ethnicity, often feel disconcerted and placed in a large context of uncertainty [11]. One can ask if they do not experience *on the contrary* difficulty using with these *foreign* patients the representativeness heuristic which usually allows them to make a given patient resemble the "class" of patients with which they feel familiar.

2. **Availability heuristic**: here, individuals associate the frequency of an event to the ease with which it can come to their mind; indeed, one remembers frequent events more easily. But here also, this can be a source of bias: one remembers

a disease more easily if one has recently seen a case; this does not increase however the frequency of the disease. Later we will consider in detail the effects of emotions as a source of cognitive biases. Yet emotions intervene powerfully in phenomena of memorization. One may easily remember a side effect which occurred following the implementation of a treatment, and, we will come back to this, one understands that this could be a source of clinical inertia.

3. **Adjustment heuristic and anchoring effects**: as we have seen, Bayes' theorem predicts that the acquisition of new information modifies the idea we have of the likelihood of an event. Nevertheless, this adjustment does not always take place, due to an "anchoring effect" linked to a saturation of reasoning possibilities, which therefore introduces a bias. A classic example illustrating the bias linked to anchoring is that given by Tversky and Kahneman [6]. Two groups of students are asked to quickly estimate the value of the products $8 \times 7 \times 6 \times 5 \times 4 \times 3 \times 2 \times 1$, or $1 \times 2 \times 3 \times 4 \times 5 \times 6 \times 7 \times 8$. They only have the time to perform a few stages of calculation and must then estimate the result through extrapolation or adjustment. The anchoring effect is conveyed by the fact that in the first case, extrapolation gives a median estimation of 2,250 and in the second case of 512 (the exact value is 40,320).

Here again, one understands that use of this heuristic can give results which are contrary to the predictions of Bayes' theorem. It tells us in fact that each new piece of information must bring about an adjustment of the idea that we have of the likelihood of occurrence of a certain event, passing from a pre-information probability to a post-information probability. Through saturation of the mind, the anchoring effect blocks our abilities of adjustment at a certain point.

## Sources of Bias in Decisions Under Risk

Kahneman and Tversky have also shown in their Prospect Theory [12] that, in decisions comprising a risk, human judgment could be subject to biases.

1. **Risk aversion**: when individuals have the choice between either receiving, for certain, $800, or taking part in a bet which presents an 85 % chance of winning $1,000, most people prefer the first alternative. Yet the expected utility in the second case is $0.85 \times 1,000 + 0.15 \times 0 = \$850$. This preference for the certain gain is an example of risk aversion. Conversely, if one offers individuals a choice between either a certain loss of $800, or to take part in a bet where there is 85 % chance of losing $1,000, most people prefer the uncertain bet, even though here also, the expected loss in the case of the bet is $850: there is therefore on the contrary, in the case of losses, a preference for risk. This effect of risk aversion manifests itself also through the fact that the degree of aversion for a loss, for example of $100, is significantly greater than the degree of attraction for a gain of the same magnitude.

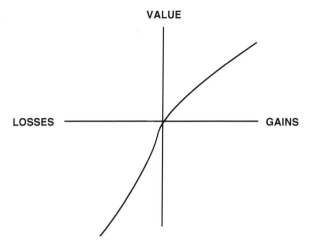

**Fig. 6.2** The utility function (From Ref. [12], reproduced with the permission of the Econometry Society)

This led Kahneman and Tversky to propose that the utility function is concave for gains (it saturates quickly) and convex for losses (Fig. 6.2), with a steeper slope for losses than for gains: the more one loses, the more one is unhappy; the more one wins, the more one is happy, but with a saturation effect, and one hates losing more than one loves winning.

This concept of risk aversion, whose importance we will see later when we consider the role of emotions in medical decisions, also explains the effect of the way in which we state a problem (framing effect).

2. **The effect of framing of a problem**: the way of asking the question, that is to say the type of statement it is made up of, intervenes in the way it is answered. For example, let's suppose that a country must cope with an epidemic that is expected to kill 600 people. In statement 1 of the problem, one proposes two programs: with program A, 200 people will be saved; if program B is adopted, there is a one in 3 chance that all 600 people are saved, and a two in three chance that nobody is saved. In this first statement of the problem, the reference point is that there is a risk of having 600 deaths; given the phenomenon of risk aversion, most people questioned prefer the solution which saves for certain 200 people over that of the bet which offers a one in three chance of saving 600 people.

In statement 2 of the problem, the solutions are presented differently: with program C, 400 people must die, while if program D is adopted, there is a one in 3 chance that nobody will die and a two in three chance that all 600 people will die. Here, the framing of the problem consists of imagining a reference state where nobody dies. With this frame, on the contrary, most people questioned prefer the bet situation.

This influence of framing of the problem, that is to say the way of presenting a choice, either in terms of risk of survival, or in terms of risk of death, has been clearly demonstrated in the case of patient choice between radiation therapy and surgery for lung cancer [13].

## Heuristics Are Necessary and Do Not Necessarily Have an Adverse Effect

Heuristics are not just mental short-cuts that allow us to reason because the capacity of our reasoning is limited. Another reason to use heuristics is that the problem posed cannot be put in the form of a decision tree; or else, the level of uncertainty cannot be quantified, or else, the targets are ambiguous. In fact, by allowing us to not have to consider all the possibilities, heuristics give us the possibility to avoid overly long hesitations. At times, they alone can be used – we then say that we must use our intuition.

Therefore one must not see in the existence of heuristics an inevitable source of bias and error, and one can find in the article by Wegwarth et al. a critical analysis of heuristics, showing that they are neither "good" nor "bad" and that an adapted use of heuristics can even be beneficial [14]. One must therefore rather see in heuristics one of the properties of human reasoning which allows it to function, but which, due to their existence, also open the door to the occurrence of bias: beware of your first impression, it's usually right, stated Talleyrand, perhaps praising thus the positive effect of a typical heuristic!

We will see later that the same is true of emotions: they are part of our mental life and in fact promote the power of our cognition, even if they can also distort our judgment. One can what's more imagine, from an evolutionary point of view, that the positive aspect of heuristics (allowing us to make decisions rapidly) and emotions (allowing us, for example, to detect the presence of a predator and to flee in time) explains that they were developed to such an extent within our mental life.

## Heuristics, Principles of Evidence-Based Medicine, and Medical Behavior: Coming Back to Clinical Inertia

Several publications have studied the application of these general psychological notions to the mental mechanisms which preside over medical decisions [15–17]. These analyses show that clinicians do not always apply, far from it, Bayesian type reasoning, which is at the base of Evidence-Based Medicine, but in fact more often call upon heuristics. Yet, we have seen that though the latter, as mental short-cuts, allow for quick decision making, they present risks of bias [18].

In other words, it may occur that when physicians use their *medical reason*, they do not have access to basically Bayesian type statistical reasoning, which represents the essence of the word "based" in the expression "Evidence-Based Medicine". *Medical reason* is instead based on unconventional modes of reasoning simpler and quicker to use which are heuristics, with their risk of bias. By bringing up to date this discordance between the *rationality* of Evidence-Based Medicine, based on data established in studies *carried out if possible without bias*, and what we have called *medical reason*, we have perhaps put a finger on a general conceptual explanation of the phenomenon of clinical inertia.

Curiously, few publications explicitly make the link between the use of heuristics, with the risk of bias derived from them, and lack of compliance with guidelines which characterizes clinical inertia. Redelmeier et al. showed on an enormous database (1,344,145 patients treated in Ontario) that patients with chronic diseases, for example diabetes, less often receive hormone replacement therapy; that patients with emphysema less often receive cholesterol lowering treatment, and that psychotic patients less often receive treatment for polyarthritis. They evoke the possibility that physicians fall prey to the heuristic which falsely suggests that it is unlikely that a given patient has two diseases (this is the *"gambler's fallacy"*, which thinks that after an unfortunate event, statistically, follows a fortunate event, this heuristic being reinforced by that of *"Occam's razor"* which recommends trying to use the simplest explanation to account for all the observed evidence) [19]. Yet, we know well that "one train may hide another"!

The study of the compliance of 25 physicians with guidelines regarding prescription of nonsteroidal anti-inflammatory drugs [20] implicitly revealed the intervention of heuristics, apart from the barriers to their implementation which we have evoked extensively in the previous chapters (lack of familiarity with guidelines, suspicion regarding the role of the pharmaceutical industry, impression that guidelines are not "evidence-based" in a sufficiently solid way, etc.). Thus, in this study, in all the physicians questioned, personal experience of positive or adverse events relating to use of a nonsteroidal anti-inflammatory drug had had an impact on compliance with guidelines: a single negative event was sufficient to have a lasting effect (availability heuristic), while positive results reinforced usual practices without taking into account the actual prevalence of side effects. In fact, when we will tackle the role of emotions in medical decisions, we will understand how the involvement of this type of heuristic undoubtedly represents a major cause of clinical inertia.

Finally one should cite the two significant publications by Richard Miles [21, 22] on the phenomena of clinical inertia which he observed in the retirement home that he directs, in the following fields: treatment of osteoporosis, prescription of anticoagulants, use of statins, performance of echocardiogram, treatment of dementia. In his two publications, the author explicitly presents a precise taxonomic description of the types of heuristics encountered in these different diseases, which result, to adopt the title of one of his articles, in a *nullification* of Evidence-Based Medicine in the retirement home. Miles suggests that this nullification is not due, on the part of the physicians, to ignorance of guidelines or lack of concern regarding patients, but to a lack of awareness of the many biases which can result from the use of judgment heuristics in the management of elderly patients.

This significant observation should have, we will see in the following chapter, implications in terms of training of future physicians, regarding the modes of reasoning which they will use later in their medical practice.

It is a matter of first initiating them to the very nature of medical reason [23]. But it is also a matter of teaching them to make the most of the fact that it is made up of, as Pat Croskerry clearly described [24–27], two modes of thought: an analytical, largely "Bayesian" mode, but also an intuitive mode, in which heuristics intervene.

As we have seen, they must be aware of the two aspects of heuristics: that which assists in reasoning and that which is a source of bias [9, 14]. A better understanding by physicians of the functioning of what we have proposed to call in this book *their medical reason* could allow them to avoid the occurrence of certain biases which, obviously, have deleterious effects on the efficiency of care. They should also learn to recognize the role of emotions in their decisions.

## Role of Emotions in Medical Decisions

In *medical reason*, there are in fact, as in all human reason, emotions, and it is possible that they contribute to the effect of heuristics which we have mentioned above: for example, the framing heuristic, which makes it that the patient's answers to a choice are different depending on whether it was put forth in terms of death or survival, can be linked to the emotions associated with the idea of death. In fact, one must consider emotions on a much broader level, admitting that medical reason has, as all reason, (at least) two components: a component which we can call cognitive and an emotional component.

In our previous work [1], devoted to patient nonadherence, which we have linked to the philosophical concept of weakness of will or *akrasia* – I do not do what I should do, or I do what I should not do, *but, what did you expect, I can't help myself* – we had mentioned the role of emotions as possible explanation of certain nonadherent behavior, thus in accordance with the philosopher Christine Tappolet in her interpretation of *akrasia*. She proposed that emotions, in that they act by influencing the way in which we perceive the value of things (she proposes that emotions are in fact the perception of values), make intelligible actions which can be described under the generic term of weakness of will [28]: for example, the pleasure of smoking makes the fact that I smoke intelligible.

The goal of the rest of this chapter is to show how emotions can intervene in medical decisions and in the birth of clinical inertia. To introduce this development, let's cite the answers of two physicians interviewed by Summerskill and Pope, in the intention to understand why they did not intensify treatment [29]: "I know what he would want and I think that maybe influenced my judgment and I was perhaps *less coldly clinical* than I could have been." (the emphasis is ours). Another physician declared: "as I saw the panic rise in her eyes, evidence-based medicine went out of the door and reassurance was what was needed, because there was very little one could do about her and I could see her husband pleading behind, 'stop talking science and start talking something else'. So I patted her on the hand and told her all was well and it would get better in a little while."

## Emotions in Mental Life

As shown in our Fig. 6.1, page 74, emotions intervene in the birth of our actions, especially by selecting, among all the available information, and emphasizing some of it [30], thus helping to avoid the pressure to choose from an overflow of information that would be paralyzing. Through this "salience" effect, they intervene what's more in the phenomena of memorization.

This major, *positive*, role of emotions in the decision making process [31] is suggested by clinical observations, especially by Antonio Damasio, whose book, *Descartes' Error. Emotions, Reason and the Human Brain* is rightly famous, on patients having lesions in the ventromedial prefrontal cortex, in whom one notes a decrease both in the capacity to feel emotions and to make decisions [32]. Damasio introduces his concept of *"somatic marker"*: the orbitofrontal cortex associates emotional sensations with a *stimulus*; it registers this relationship and will be able to reactivate the emotional sensations during a subsequent encounter with the stimulus; these somatic markers therefore allow the individual to take into consideration her previous encounters with stimuli and to draw upon this for the carrying out of her choices and her action plans.

Here, this is the positive role of emotions, which save us, by selecting them, from having to consider too many arguments, which would lead us to never-ending procrastination. Indeed, the role of emotions in this selection appears in the definition given by Pierre Livet and in the role which he attributes them in the *revision* of mental states: emotions are born of the observation of a difference between what we think of the state of the world and what we observe (for example, I thought all was tranquil in the forest, seeing a snake brings about the appearance of fright) and they lead to a revision of what we think [3].

## Emotions in Medical Decisions

Croskerry et al. recently reviewed the different aspects of the role of emotions in care, how they can, through diverse mechanisms, have an impact on the safety of patients [33]. Even in the case of emergency medicine [24, 25], the skills of the physician involve three fields of expertise: not only procedural (for example knowing how to perform a lumbar puncture), but also cognitive (knowing how to make a diagnosis, ask for the appropriate lab tests, offer a treatment based on the best data available), and emotional. This last field of expertise consists, for the physician, of recognizing her emotions, and, if possible, being able to limit their effects. Croskerry et al. note that this last field is underexplored and that the errors derived from it are considerably less visible than those in the procedural or cognitive fields of expertise [24–27]. What's more not all emotions have a negative role, and it was recently proposed that having a "gut feeling" could intervene as a positive element in medical decisions due to its quick nature (I don't know why, I have the feeling that there is something seriously wrong and I have the patient hospitalized), to the same extent as the more cognitive processes of decision making and problem solving [34].

We have seen above how the cognitive decision making process can be affected by the use of different heuristics, these quick procedures presenting the risk of leading to a bias. Yet there are also emotional heuristics which intervene in *medical reason* and which can have a negative effect on medical decisions. Croskerry et al. cite thus:

1. **"ego bias"**, the tendency to underestimate one's own errors (we recall that Phillips clearly stated in his description of clinical inertia [35] that one of its causes was denial of the existence of the phenomenon);
2. **"anticipated regret"** (we also spoke of *chagrin*), which consists of not doing something whose outcome one thinks presents a risk, in fact in order to not experience regret afterwards – we will come back later in detail to this chagrin heuristic since it is fundamental in explaining clinical inertia;
3. **"outcome bias"**, which consists of deciding based on the expected result, by giving preference to decisions which lead to results which are to our advantage;
4. **"status quo bias"**, to which we will come back to also at the end of this chapter, which consists of perpetuating the current situation to avoid the emotional discomfort of new situations– therefore leading to inertia.

## Emotions and Cognition: Two Components of Reason

Thus, what was described by the name of affect heuristics [36] can certainly increase the effectiveness of medical reason (we have cited the quick effect of gut feelings, which make us feel for example that there is an urgent problem to resolve) but can also decrease it: they seem therefore to have a positive and negative effect on the effectiveness of our behavior. In such a conception of mental life, *medical reason* would therefore be essentially of a cognitive nature, being in a way modulated by the intervention of emotions.

In what follows, we will present another conception of mental life, in the form of two psychological models connecting emotions and behavior and proposing that reason has in fact two components, cognitive and emotional. We will insist upon the importance, among the negative emotions, of regret. We will show how these models can be relevant in our search for the comprehension of, that is to say *the explanation in general* of, the clinical inertia phenomenon. We will therefore propose a description of clinical inertia in terms of the psychology of the *status quo*, which gave the title to this chapter: to do…*or not to do*.

## Emotions as Notification of the Feeling of Risk

As we have seen, all medical decisions can be considered as taking a risk, for a variety of reasons, linked both to the variability of living phenomena and the fact that one does not know the result of a treatment until after the fact, as in the experiments of Schrödinger's cat and Einstein's boxes: it is only after the treatment has been instituted and that one sees the patient again, that one will, on an individual basis, know the result. The predictions from clinical trials, as has been strongly insisted upon, in fact have only a strictly statistical value.

Loewenstein et al. [37] noted that classic models of decision in conditions of risk are essentially of a "consequentialist" type, meaning by this that individuals make

Emotions and Cognition: Two Components of Reason

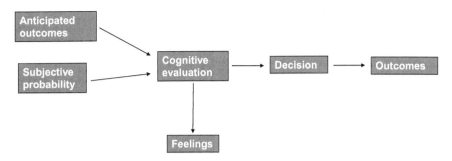

**Fig. 6.3** Consequentialist model of decision making (From Ref. [37], reproduced with permission of the American Psychological Association, © 2001)

their decision by assessing the consequences of their choice. One can note that this is typically the case of therapeutic choice, as described in Fig. 5.4 of Chap. 5, page 56.

More generally, in these classic models of rational choice, emotions can be regarded as epiphenomena (Fig. 6.3).

In their article, Loewenstein et al. propose first to distinguish what they call anticipatory emotions and anticipated emotions. Anticipatory emotions are immediate affects, visceral, for example fear, anxiety, terror, which one feels at the moment of preparing to carry out an action which presents a risk. Anticipated emotions are not felt immediately, but are those that one imagines that one may feel as a consequence of the decision: these can be positive emotions such as pride or joy, or negative, such as regret or disappointment. It is possible to integrate these anticipated emotions into a consequentialist model, such as the one presented in Fig. 6.3. It suffices to say that, among the anticipated results, the individual cognitively evaluates the anticipated emotion which she may feel, this also being part of what was placed in the "box" representing in this figure the outcome of the decision.

Nevertheless, with the goal of integrating both types of emotions, anticipatory and anticipated, into a model of decision making within the context of risk, the authors proposed a hypothesis, which they call "the risk-as-feelings hypothesis": individuals cognitively evaluate the alternatives of the choice at risk, as in the traditional model, while largely taking into account the desirability and the probability of occurrence of the result (typically the "expected utility" which we have seen previously). This cognitive evaluation has consequences, triggering emotions which interact with the results of the cognitive evaluation (Fig. 6.4).

But what's more, one sees in this figure that "feelings" can also be triggered noncognitively, quickly, based on the context, put in the box on the lower left in this figure. This is the intervention of our gut feelings which we have mentioned above. One sees also that the authors deliberately replaced the word "decision" in the previous figure by the word "behavior": it can in fact happen that what we do under the influence of these intense feelings (the agoraphobic who remains frozen in place under the influence of panic) may not be assimilated into a decision. Moreover, they insist upon the contribution of this model, for example when it is compared to other hypotheses such as those of "somatic markers" proposed by Damasio or

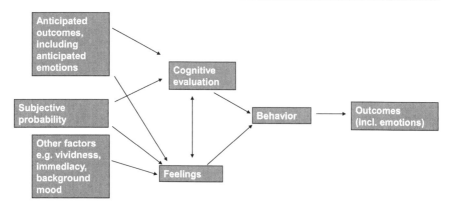

**Fig. 6.4** The "risk-as-feelings" hypothesis by Loewenstein et al., from Ref. [37], reproduced with permission of the American Psychological Association, © 2001

the hypothesis of affect heuristics which we have mentioned above, which came to disrupt the results of cognitive deliberation.

In this model of "risk-as feelings" proposed by Loewenstein et al., this is indeed a description of *reason*, having two distinct paths which can possibly be contradictory. They cite the distinction between emotion and cognition proposed by Zajonc in his chapter on emotions in the *Handbook of Social Psychology* (1998), proposing that emotions are there to help people to distinguish approach from avoidance, while cognition helps them essentially to distinguish true from false. Nevertheless, this distinction between emotion and cognition might in fact be just an appearance: some see in emotions a true cognition [38].

## Relationship Between Emotions and Behavior: Rather Than Causation, a Feedback Dynamic

In the previous model, the arrow connecting "feelings" and behavior appears to give emotions a causal effect. Baumeister et al. [39] note that this idea has the advantage of being intuitive (my fear *caused my* flight), but it encounters several objections: for example, it is primarily negative emotions (fear, hatred etc.) that appear to have this effect. Moreover, how can emotions which occur after the fact cause behavior? What of those emotions that one feels and that do not lead to action? If emotions cause behavior that is often disastrous for the individual, how were these mental processes that are so general conserved by evolution?

Based on this critique, Baumeister et al. proposed another model in which emotions influence behavior in a feedback type system: in this model also, they make the distinction between immediate emotions and anticipated emotions. They give the following example: someone has a behavior which hurts a friend. She feels after the fact a feeling of guilt. This feeling leads the individual to reflect on what she might have done wrong and how to prevent this from happening again. On the next occasion, a brief recollection of this feeling of guilt occurs as a flash, helping the individual to avoid this behavior which could hurt friends, and to avoid having the feeling of guilt again. In fact, what recollection of the emotion does, is confirm (if the emotion was positive – let's take for example the feeling of pride in the case where the action on the contrary benefitted the friend) or revise (if it was negative) the cognitive reasoning which leads to action, which are in general rules of the type "if – then" (example: if she says this, then I will answer that): the next time that she will be tempted to act in the same way and to apply this rule, resurgence of the affect will be activated automatically, warning the individual that she should not repeat the same error. It appears therefore in this model that the role of emotions, contrary to what one believes intuitively, is not to cause behavior, but to shape the cognitive process.

In this model, anticipated emotions play a major role. Emotional residues are there to remind me that when I had the inappropriate behavior, I experienced regret, shame, etc. I find myself in an identical situation: to avoid this displeasure, I modify my rules of behavior. Baumeister et al. elegantly note that one can understand, within the context of this theory, why one cannot control one's emotions: you cannot control them, *because the role of emotions is precisely to control you*; emotions represent a feedback system whose goal is to promote learning and the control of behavior.

One can give an illustration of the importance of anticipated emotions by using the example reported by Baumeister et al.: it is known that sadness leads people to eat more, because they think that after having eaten, they will feel less sad. In an experimental context, a feeling of sadness was induced in volunteers; indeed, it was observed that they ate more cookies. But this effect did not take place if the experiment's subjects had been told that they would not feel better after having eaten: thus, sadness induces the behavior only if the subject can anticipate that the behavior will have a happy emotional effect.

## Chagrin and Regret: Application to the Issue of Clinical Inertia

Among these anticipated emotions, one must emphasize regret. Avoidance of regret is a powerful factor in remodeling our behavior, and its cerebral mechanisms are starting to be studied [40]. One can take two examples: (1) how is it that one regrets more having "missed one's train" by 3 min than by half an hour? One should expect the opposite effect: if I missed it by half an hour, I am more at fault. In fact, the more powerful effect of regret in the case of the train "just missed" is due to the fact that it is easy to avoid this from occurring: the next time, I'll avoid drinking the extra cup of coffee before leaving home. It is therefore good that I am reminded of this in a particularly intense way the next time I have to take the train: this is why the emotion felt is stronger; it could have more of an educational effect [41]. (2) A study consisted of offering people to buy a ski-lift pass, which is normally worth 100€, for the sum of either 40€ or 80€. They decline. The following week, it is offered to them for 90€, which is again less expensive than the true value of the pass, but which represents less of a "good deal". Those who had refused to buy it at 40€ are less likely to buy it, in fact *to avoid the feeling of regret* of having missed a good opportunity the previous week, that is to say to avoid a displeasure [42].

In 1985, at the time where Evidence-Based Medicine was establishing itself, Feinstein published an article criticizing the use of mathematical estimations of "expected utilities" when the physician finds herself faced with a choice whose result she doesn't know in advance. He proposed that physicians use in fact a much simpler means of reasoning, asking themselves: between the two alternatives of a choice at risk, if the choice that I make turns out to be wrong, which is the alternative that will cause me the most "*chagrin*", or regret [43].

More precisely, I can choose between prescribing a treatment (the active option) or I can do nothing (the passive option). In general, the active option has a greater chance of improving the patient's condition, but it also presents more risk than the passive option, or rather, it's a risk that I would make her take, while the side effects of the passive option are those of the disease. If I choose the active option and if it is successful, the pleasure will be great. The same is true if I choose the passive option, if it turns out that I was right. In both cases, either I got lucky, or I showed good judgment.

Of course, we seek pleasure and wish to avoid pain, but, as we have seen above (Kahneman and Tversky Prospect Theory), our aversion for losses is significantly greater than our attraction for gains. It is therefore especially after a failure that we think. A bad result occurs when, after choice of the active option, an adverse event occurs (due to the disease or the treatment) or when it occurs when one had chosen the passive option. Seen retrospectively, each of these adverse effects can be due to bad luck, but one of the two or both cause me chagrin. I will choose the option which avoids or minimizes this retrospective chagrin. This is the reason, Feinstein states, why physicians often prefer to appear pessimistic with patients: they fear that an unfortunate event will occur when they have announced a happy outcome – the chagrin would be even greater.

Consequently, if we take Fig. 6.4, by specifying that the anticipated emotion is regret (what Feinstein calls chagrin), and that one wishes to avoid it, this mechanism should protect us against clinical inertia: I should prescribe the treatment to avoid having to regret the consequences of my inaction. But since there are reasons both for and against intensifying or not intensifying the treatment, in fact, application of the model by Feinstein predicts that one can give the favor to the behavior of clinical inertia. Indeed, it's here that heuristics exert their disruptive effect: one of them stipulates, we have seen, that we regret more losses which occur due to our action than those which are the consequence of our inaction – we prefer to commit an error of omission (clinical inertia) than an error of commission; this is undoubtedly due to the availability heuristic, which makes it that we estimate the probability of occurrence of an event based on the ease with which we remember it; yet we remember with particular intensity iatrogenic events for which we are responsible: it may be easier to retrieve examples of side effects due to the greater power of bad events over good ones on learning processes [44].

We can now propose an explanation of physicians' behavior when faced with the prescription of anticoagulants in embolic event prevention in atrial fibrillation: we had cited the study by Choudhry et al. [45] showing that prescriptions of anticoagulant decreased after the occurrence of an hemorrhagic stroke (a complication of the treatment seen as an error of commission), but did not increase after an embolic event which occurred in untreated patients (a complication that could be interpreted as the consequences of the behavior of clinical inertia, seen as an error of omission).

We had cited, in the chapter describing different models of clinical inertia, the Regulatory Focus Theory by Higgins [46], describing two possible orientations of individuals when they set themselves an objective, identifying with either a promotion or a prevention "focus". They differ in their awareness, in the first, to a choice between gain and non-gain, and in the second, to a choice between loss and non-loss. Veazie [47] proposed that a promotion focus focuses the attention of the physician on the advantages of a treatment while a prevention focus shows her in particular the inconveniences of its side effects. The risk aversion heuristic can reinforce the fact that the avoidance of pain which characterizes a prevention focus could be conceptually associated with clinical inertia.

Emotions could intervene in this model: Higgins et al. showed in empirical trials that the strength of the orientation (whether it be of a promotion or prevention type) was associated with the intensity of the emotions felt when the goal that one set is reached [48].

## Emotions in the Interaction Between Physician and Patient, and in the Relationship Between Clinical Inertia and Nonadherence

Intervention of anticipated emotions in *medical reason*, such as it can be described in the models which have just been described, can also allow one to understand certain risk behaviors, including patient nonadherence (Fig. 6.5).

Take the example of the choice between patient adherence (for example abstaining from smoking) and nonadherence, in this example smoking. Present emotions are the pleasure of smoking. Anticipated emotions are the pleasure of having smoked or regret. The subject will smoke if she gives priority to pleasure over

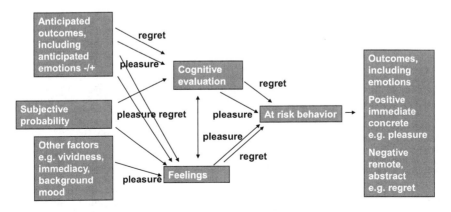

**Fig. 6.5** from the patients' side, patient nonadherence seen as the consequence of *inoperant regret*

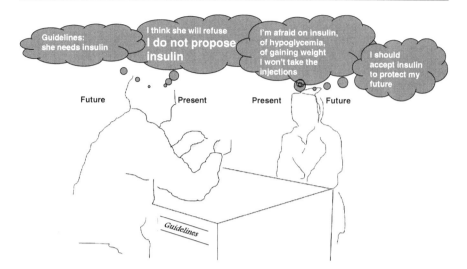

**Fig. 6.6** Clinical Inertia as clinical myopia, giving priority to immediate emotions

avoidance of regret, in other words *if regret becomes inoperant*. In the case of the accomplishment of prevention actions for weight control (physical activity, following of dietary guidelines), Bagozzi et al. clearly demonstrated the role of anticipated emotions [49]. Incidentally, we think that these concepts of use of anticipated emotions should be used more to motivate patients to seek treatment.

It appears thus that the same type of model can be used to represent both physician and patient *medical reason*, with its two components, cognitive (reasoning, itself subjected to the biases of heuristics) and emotional, leading the physician to be inert or not and the patient to be adherent or not. One notes in the previous figure regarding patient nonadherence that anticipated emotions were distinguished as positive emotions, which are concrete and immediate, such as pleasure, and as negative emotions, which are abstract and regarding the future, such as regret. The same type of distinction could be made in the case of clinical inertia. This is why we have suggested to see in physician clinical inertia and patient nonadherence a clinical myopia [4]: we have proposed in our book *Une Théorie du soin, souci et amour face à la maladie* to consider that clinical inertia could represent a side effect of a misuse by the physician of her empathic desire to acknowledge the emotions of her patient [50], this hypothesis being described in detail in a chapter of our book *The Mental Mechanisms of Patient Adherence to Long Term Therapies, Mind and Care* [1].

Figure 6.6 attempts in fact to represent the interrelationship of an emotional nature between the two protagonists of care, giving priority to immediate emotions over concerns regarding the future.

This is indeed a misuse of empathy if one recalls the classic definition given by Carl Rogers [51]: "The state of empathy, or being empathic, is to perceive the internal frame of reference of another with accuracy and with the emotional components and meanings which pertain thereto as if one were the person, but without ever losing the 'as if' condition. Thus it means to sense the hurt or the pleasure of another as he senses it and to perceive the causes thereof as he perceives them, but without ever losing the recognition that it is as if I were hurt or pleased and so forth. If this 'as if' quality is lost, then the state is one of identification." Lauren Wispé proposed to see here the difference between empathy and sympathy, which is emotional identification [52]. The misuse consists of the omission of the last clause: the physician should remember that she is still the physician and that her role as physician is to give priority to the future. One can imagine that this omission is the consequence of a bias introduced into the *medical reason* of the physician by one or undoubtedly several of the heuristics which we have mentioned in this chapter.

## ...Or Not to Do: Psychology of the Status Quo and the Difficulty of Making a Decision

Finally, how is it that, so often, we prefer the *status quo*? If we admit that clinical inertia consists of not doing something (prescribe, intensify a treatment) that one thinks one should have done, this type of behavior, which appears to resemble a weakness of will, can in fact be situated at several levels of decision making. In general, it is possible to distinguish several types of "weakness of will" or *akrasia* [53]: there is the inability to take action (last-ditch *akrasia*), the inability to carry out the action that we think is the best (conventional *akrasia*), finally *the inability to generate options*, often described by philosophers under the term of accidie, sometimes referred to as laziness or indolence (we can think of the idleness of Oblomov, hero of the novel by Gontcharov).

Clinical inertia seen as a case of conventional *akrasia* can fall within the same mechanisms which lead to patient nonadherence, such as we have analyzed it in our book on the mechanisms of patient adherence [1] and we have already mentioned a few of these mechanisms, in particular the intervention of emotions. Here we wish to focus on the last type of weakness of will, that in which the physician *avoids making the decision*. This type of behavior, which leads one to do nothing, was the subject (of course, in general and not dedicated to the specific problem of clinical inertia) of a detailed review by Anderson, entitled *The psychology of doing nothing* [54].

In this article, the author described several types of decision avoidance: preference for the *status quo*, omission, postponement. He proposes a "rational-emotional" type psychological model very close to those which we have seen previously, involving in particular the role of uncertainty, of regret as an anticipated emotion (the author puts another emotion on the same level which could be relevant to the issue of clinical inertia, fear of blame), of risk aversion, finally a notion that is obviously interesting for our subject: *the difficulty of making a decision*.

For Anderson, the fact that one finds it *difficult* to make a decision is not equivalent to a feeling of uncertainty. He gives as example the student who has forgotten her pencil the day of the test, and must choose between two types of pen offered to her; she does not know which is the best but will not find it difficult to make a decision; neither is a difficult decision one in which one feels intense emotions: the virologist, who is faced with an extremely serious epidemic and who must decide between two treatments of the same cost but where one will save 1.5 % and the other 4 % of the population, is placed in a highly emotional situation but will not find it difficult to make a decision. A difficult decision can what's more be seen even in the absence of uncertainty or emotion, although uncertainty and emotions are associated with the difficulty of the decision.

Among the many factors which can lead to rendering a decision difficult and lead to inaction *in general*, discussed by Anderson in his review, one can retain the following: the difficulty of adopting a clear strategy *due to lack of time*, getting hung up on the details, the multiplicity of options, uncertainty regarding preferences, the fact that the choice is poorly defined, the greater or lesser attractiveness of different options, perhaps the personality of the agent, even her culture.

It is interesting to note that we find determinants that we have noted throughout our analysis of clinical inertia: of course, uncertainty (uncertainty regarding the elevated nature of blood pressure readings is of course but one of the elements of a much more general concept), but also, simply, *lack of time*, which can lead to clinical inertia in appointments that are too short, especially when the physician must treat a "competing demand" [55].

*
* *

The purpose of this *critique of medical reason* was to show that what one calls clinical inertia can in part be explained by using general hypotheses made by psychologists and economists with the goal of exploring the birth of human behavior. These hypotheses can allow one to understand how the mental mechanisms which govern "medical reason" at times lead patients to not be adherent to physicians' guidelines and physicians to not follow clinical practice guidelines: one is forced to consider *the individual psychology* of physicians to understand why it occurs that they do not apply the guidelines, just as one must consider that of the patient to understand why she cannot be adherent with a prescription which, in general, is beneficial.

Regarding Evidence-Based Medicine, one insists upon the need to take into account *the patient as an individual* on whom one wishes to apply a clinical practice guideline. The surprise felt when one discovers the frequency of clinical inertia comes perhaps from the fact that one has the tendency to forget that clinical practice guidelines will ultimately be applied by physicians *who are also human beings*, and whose *medical reason* is not molded on the pure rationality of Evidence-Based Medicine: like all human actions, medical practice presents the risk of encountering many cognitive biases and its rationality is based on two components, one part rational and one part emotional.

Noting that in clinical trials one manages, through certain methods, to minimize patient nonadherence and physician clinical inertia, one can propose that the physician, in her daily practice, could draw upon this [56]: of course, the physician, when she treats a patient, could find an advantage to imposing on herself the rigor to which are subjected the physicians who perform a clinical trial. One must nevertheless not forget the fundamental difference between the clinical trial and care. The first is made to demonstrate something, and it must therefore use a method which minimizes bias; it's the investigator who decides on the question and who chooses patients as "material" to answer it, defining the inclusion and exclusion criteria etc. Care is made to treat a patient; here, there is no inclusion or exclusion criterion, since it's the patient who asks the question that the physician will attempt to answer. Neither the patient's question, nor the physician's answer can be written in advance, as is the protocol of the clinical trial. And one will find both in the way, for the one, to ask the question, and for the other, to answer it, the impact of emotions and heuristics.

In fact, in care, in general there is not only one *question* – there are always several – and, rather than questions, it's the *situation* which one must speak of. Again one measures here the fact that Evidence-Based Medicine, on the one side, and daily medical practice, on the other, are based on *categorically* different dynamics.

*

* *

The fact remains that the behavior of nonadherence on the part of the patient, and clinical inertia on the part of the health care provider, even if they are therefore understandable, have at times deleterious effects which could have been avoided and this is why it is often said that it would be important to improve patient adherence and overcome physician clinical inertia. We are speaking of course here of *true* clinical inertia, that which cannot be justified, not of carefully thought out inaction of the physician who thinks that she should not apply the guideline to the patient in front of her.

Prevention of this "true" clinical inertia can pass through organizational or technical type methods, but it should also take into account *medical reason*, such as we have attempted to describe it, in all its complexity. How can one overcome this true clinical inertia by reconciling the two dynamics of the rationality of Evidence-Based Medicine and the medical reason of the physician: this is the subject of the last chapter of this book.

---

## References

1. Reach G. The mental mechanisms of patient adherence to long term therapies, mind and care, Foreword by Pascal Engel, "Philosophy and Medicine" series, Springer, forthcoming.
2. Searle J. L'Intentionalité, Editions de Minuit, 1985.
3. Livet P. Émotions et rationalité morale, P.U.F., Collection Sociologies, 2002.
4. Reach G. Patient nonadherence and healthcare-provider inertia are clinical myopia. Diabetes Metab. 2008;34:382–5.
5. Gabbay J, le May A. Evidence based guidelines or collectively constructed "mindlines"? Ethnographic study of knowledge management in primary care. BMJ. 2004;329:1013–7.
6. Kahneman D, Tversky A. Choices, values and frames. In: Kahneman D, Tversky A, editors. Choices, values and frames. Cambridge, UK: Cambridge University Press; 2000. p. 1–16.

7. Gilovich T, Griffin D. Introduction –Heuristics and biases: then and now. In: Gilovich T, Griffin D, Kahnneman D, editors. Heuristics and biases. The psychology of intuitive judgment. New York/Cambridge, UK: Cambridge University Press; 2002. p. 1–2.
8. Tversky A, Kahneman D. Judgment under uncertainty: heuristics and biases. Science. 1974;185:1124–31.
9. Croskerry P. The cognitive imperative: thinking about how we think. Acad Emerg Med. 2000;7:1223–31.
10. Payne VL, Crowley RS. Assessing use of cognitive heuristic representativeness in clinical reasoning. In: AMIA 2008 symposium proceedings. AMIA Symposium, American Medical Informatics Association. 2008. p. 571–5.
11. Kai J, Beavan J, Faull C, Lynne D, Gill P, Beighton A. Professional uncertainty and disempowerment responding to ethnic diversity in health care: a qualitative study. PLoS Med. 2007;4:1766–75.
12. Kahneman D, Tversky A. Prospect theory: an analysis of decision under risk. Econometrica. 1979;47:263–92.
13. McNeil BJ, Pauker SG, Sox Jr HC, Tversky A. On the elicitation of preferences for alternative therapies. N Engl J Med. 1982;306:1259–62.
14. Wegwarth O, Gaissmaier W, Gigerenzer G. Smart strategies for doctors and doctors-in-training: heuristics in medicine. Med Educ. 2009;43:721–8.
15. Dawson NV. Physician judgment in clinical settings: methodological influences and cognitive performances. Clin Chem. 1993;39:1468–80.
16. Bornstein BH, Emler AC. Rationality in medical decision making: a review of the literature on doctors' decision-making biases. J Eval Clin Pract. 2001;7:97–107.
17. Klein JG. Five pitfalls in decisions about diagnosis and prescribing. BMJ. 2005;330:781–3.
18. Elstein AS, Schwarz A. Clinical problem solving and diagnostic decision making: selective review of the cognitive literature. BMJ. 2002;324:729–32.
19. Redelmeier DA, Tan SH, Booth GL. The treatment of unrelated disorders in patients with chronic medical diseases. N Engl J Med. 1998;338:1516–20.
20. Cavazos JM, Naik AD, Woofter A, Abraham S. Barriers to physician adherence to nonsteroidal anti-inflammatory drug guidelines: a qualitative study. Aliment Pharmacol Ther. 2008;28:789–98.
21. Miles RW. Fallacious reasoning and complexity as route causes of clinical inertia. J Am Med Dir Assoc. 2007;8:349–54.
22. Miles RW. Cognitive bias and planning error: nullification of EBM in the nursing home. J Am Med Dir Assoc. 2010;11:194–203.
23. Masquelet AC. Le Raisonnement médical. P.U.F. "Que sais-je?", Paris, 2006.
24. Croskerry P. A universal model of diagnostic reasoning. Acad Med. 2009;84:1022–8.
25. Croskerry P, Nimmo GR. Better clinical decision making and reducing diagnostic error. J R Coll Physicians Edinb. 2011;41:155–62.
26. Croskerry P. From mindless to mindful practice–cognitive bias and clinical decision making. N Engl J Med. 2013;368:2445–8.
27. Croskerry P, Singhal G, Mamede S. Cognitive debiasing 1: origins of bias and theory of debiasing. BMJ Qual Saf. 2013;22 Suppl 2:ii58–64.
28. Tappolet C. Emotions and the intelligibility of akratic actions. In: Stroud S, Tappolet C, editors. Weakness of will and practical irrationality. Clarendon Press: Oxford; 2003. p. 97–120.
29. Summerskill WSM, Pope C. I saw the panic rise in her eyes, and evidence-based medicine went out of the door. An exploratory qualitative study of the barriers to secondary prevention in the management of coronary heart disease. Fam Pract. 2002;19:605–10.
30. de Souza R. The rationality of emotion. Cambridge: MIT Press; 1987. p. 195–8.
31. Berthoz A. La Décision, Editions Odile Jacob, 2002.
32. Damasio AR. Descartes' error. Emotions, reason and the human brain. New York: G. P. Putnam's Sons; 1994.

# References

33. Croskerry P, Abbass A, Wu AW. Emotional influences in patient safety. J Patient Saf. 2010;6:199–205.
34. Stolper E, Van de Wiel M, Van Royen P, Van Bokhoven M, Van der Weijden T, Dinant GJ. Gut feelings as a third track in general practitioners' diagnostic reasoning. J Gen Intern Med. 2011;26:197–203.
35. Phillips LS, Branch WT, Cook CB, Doyle JP, El-Kebbi IM, Gallina DL, et al. Clinical inertia. Ann Intern Med. 2001;135:825–34.
36. Slovic P, Finucane M, Peters E, MacGregor DG. The affect heuristic. In: Gilovich T, Griffin D, Kahneman D, editors. Heuristics and biases: the psychology of intuitive judgment. Cambridge, MA: Cambridge University Press; 2002. p. 397–420.
37. Loewenstein GF, Weber EU, Hsee CK, Welch N. Risk as feelings. Psychol Bull. 2001;127:267–86.
38. Oum R, Lieberman D. Emotion is cognition: an information-processing view of the mind. In: Vohs KD, Baumeister RF, Loewenstein G, editors. Do emotions help or hurt decision making. New York: Russell Sage; 2007. p. 117–32.
39. Baumeister RF, Vohs KD, DeWall CN, Zhang L. How emotion shapes behavior: feedback, anticipation, and reflexion, rather than direct causation. PSPR. 2007;11:167–203.
40. Coricelli G, Dolan RJ, Sirigu A. Brain, emotion and decision making: the paradigmatic example of regret. Trends Cogn Sci. 2007;11:258–65.
41. Kahneman D, Tversky A. The simulation heuristic. In: Kahneman D, Slovic P, Tversky A, editors. Judgment under uncertainty. New York/Cambridge, UK: Cambridge University Press; 1982. p. 201–8.
42. Tykocinski OE, Pittman TS. Product aversion following a missed opportunity: price contrast or avoidance of anticipated regret? Basic Appl Soc Psychol. 2001;23:149–56.
43. Feinstein AR. The 'chagrin factor' and qualitative decision analysis. Arch Intern Med. 1985;145:1257–9.
44. Baumeister RF, Bratslavsky E, Finkenauer C, Vohs KD. Bad is stronger than good. Rev Gen Psychol. 2001;5:323–70.
45. Choudhry NK, Anderson GM, Laupacis A, Ross-Degnan D, Normand SLT, Soumerai SB. Impact of adverse events on prescribing warfarin in patients with atrial fibrillation: matched pair analysis. BMJ. 2006;332:141–5. doi:10.1136/bmj.38698.709572.55.
46. Higgins ET. Beyond pleasure and pain. Am Psychol. 1997;52:1280–300.
47. Veazie PJ, Qian F. A role for regulatory focus in explaining and combating clinical inertia. J Eval Clin Pract. 2011;17:1147–52.
48. Higgins ET, Shah J, Friedman R. Emotional responses to goal attainment: strength of regulatory focus as moderator. J Pers Soc Psychol. 1997;72:515–25.
49. Bagozzi RP, Baumgartner H, Pieters R. Goal-directed emotions. Cogn Emotion. 1998;12:1–26.
50. Reach G. Une Théorie du soin, Souci et amour face à la maladie. Préface de Bernard Baertschi, Les Belles Lettres "Médecine et Sciences Humaines", Paris, 2010.
51. Rogers C. Psychothérapie et relations humaines, vol. 1. Louvain: Editions Universitaires; 1962. p. 197.
52. Wispé L. The distinction between sympathy and empathy: to call forth a concept, a word is needed. J Pers Soc Psychol. 1996;50:314–21.
53. Kalis A, Mojzisch A, Schweizer TS, Kaiser S. Weakness of will, akrasia, and the neuropsychiatry of decision making: an interdisciplinary perspective. Cogn Affect Behav Neurosci. 2008;8:402–17.
54. Anderson CJ. The psychology of doing nothing: forms of decision avoidance result from reason and emotion. Psychol Bull. 2003;129:139–67.
55. Parchman ML, Pugh JA, Romero RL, Bowers KW. Competing demands or clinical inertia: the case of elevated glycosylated hemoglobin. Ann Fam Med. 2007;5:196–201.
56. Jandrain BJ, Ernest PH, Radermcker RP, Scheen AJ. Stratégies pour éviter l'inertie et la non-observance dans les essais cliniques. Rev Med Liege. 2010;65:246–9.

# Overcoming *True* Clinical Inertia

**7**

**Abstract**

This chapter analyzes various approaches to overcoming true clinical inertia, that which cannot be justified. (1) Education of physicians, during their initial training and through Continuous Medical Education. (2) Facilitators: use of protocols, electronic medical records, disease management, establishment of a Coordinated Health Care Plan, use of telemedicine. (3) Strengthening the physician's motivation through incentives by health authorities (pay for performance), by peers and other healthcare professionals (pharmacists, nurses), and by patients. The physician's own self-incentive, in the form of precommitment, is analyzed in detail by calling upon concepts developed within the framework of the philosophy of mind, with a special focus on the importance of habit. (4) We insist upon the importance of the physician knowing the risks presented by the use of heuristics. (5) Finally, concerning the management of emotions, we propose the concept of emotional reversal, the physician calling on positive emotions such as pride. The best rampart against clinical inertia may well be concern for the future safety of the patient, an emotion which can be understood as the philosophic meaning of care.

In short, we have seen how knowledge and skills, beliefs, and emotions intervene in the physician's motivation to apply *or not apply* a clinical practice guideline, ultimately able to lead to the desire or lack of desire to apply the guideline. Based on these observations that may appear to be simply a truism, it is possible to construct a model allowing one to describe different possible points of impact for overcoming clinical inertia (Fig. 7.1).

(1) By "Education", we mean not only training of physicians (and future physicians) on guidelines themselves, but also on the principles of a sound use of Evidence-Based Medicine, the "titration" of treatment in the management of chronic diseases, and finally the psychology of reasoning and medical decisions,

© Springer International Publishing Switzerland 2015
G. Reach, *Clinical Inertia: A Critique of Medical Reason*,
DOI 10.1007/978-3-319-09882-1_7

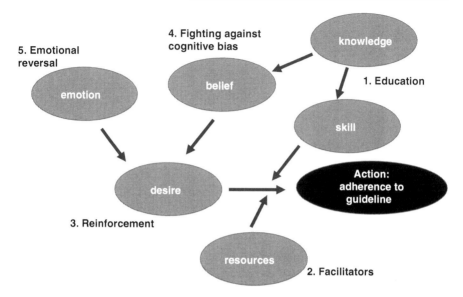

**Fig. 7.1** *Medical reason* and different points of impact of interventions aiming to overcome Clinical Inertia

such as they are outlined in this book; (2) by "Facilitator" elements, we mean the technical and human resources which will help them to apply guidelines; (3) by "Reinforcement", we mean all of the different means aiming to motivate physicians to apply the guideline; (4) we will see how it is possible to avoid certain cognitive biases; finally (5) under the term "Emotional reversal", we will particularly describe how physicians can learn the right way to make use of anticipated emotions.

## Education

### Initial Training of Physicians

One can only convince someone of the merit of something if one is oneself convinced. Regarding guidelines that have a purpose of preventing complications from diseases, the physician must therefore first herself be fully conscious of the benefit of applying, with all the limits which we have continually mentioned, certain rules of best practice to enable *herself* to actually apply them. This means that she must have a strong conscience of her role as a health care provider being responsible for the health of a patient with a chronic disease: to help her avoid long term complications and, ultimately, prolong her life; for this she must correct the modifiable risk factors, know that these pass both through prescription of a healthy lifestyle and, through a drug level, through "titration" of treatment, that is to say that often several medications are needed at the right doses to reach a preset target. Of course, one must be aware of the right use of medication, especially while remaining particularly critical

Education                                                                              99

regarding new medications and paying particular attention to the difficulty of care of patients with several diseases and "polymedicated" [1]. But neither must one say "one prescribes too many medications": it is due to medications, particularly those for diabetes, blood pressure and cholesterol that the last decades have seen an unprecedented increase in life expectancy.

The physician would be conscious of the fact that this is an often arduous path, which is the opposite of ease; that she can expect refusal from the patient and non-adherence; that she is herself at risk of the clinical inertia phenomenon. She will also know to remember the fact that her judgment can be subjected to cognitive biases or the effect of emotions: she would be aware of the existence of heuristics, with their positive aspects [2], but also as a source of bias in reasoning. Of course, we will repeat one more time, when she will apply the principles of Evidence-Based Medicine, she will do so while always asking herself the question of the appropriateness of the guideline for this particular patient and by always giving priority to her clinical judgment; but she will do so "honestly", that is to say by trying to avoid using this sound reservation as an alibi for not intensifying treatment and give in to the ease which consists of "renewing the prescription". Moreover, regarding fear of a refusal of treatment intensification on the part of the patient or of subsequent nonadherence, she should ask, regarding patient refusal, if this is not *a presupposition* as long as intensification has not been offered and explained, and regarding her possible nonadherence, again, she will know to guard against anticipating it without having actually observed it. It appears to us that this here is clearly the misuse of empathy which we have mentioned in the previous chapter, coming back to put oneself in the patient's position ("in her position", I would refuse this treatment or I would not implement it). This emotional identification can lead to clinical inertia [3].

These remarks suggest that physician training should associate with the teaching of medical knowledge, that is to say diseases and their treatment, and the Evidence which is at the base of guidelines, the way to use them, that is to say a sound practice of Evidence-Based Medicine: this involves training on the management of chronic diseases in general, on the mechanisms of medical reason and therapeutic decisions, on the phenomena of nonadherence and clinical inertia, elements which could be presented as of the start of medical studies, for example in France through the teaching of Social Sciences in the first year of the medical curriculum [4].

## Continuing Medical Education

Subsequently, the role of Continuing Medical Education throughout the physician's professional life will be important, just as is participation at conventions and post-graduate training sessions. We have cited a publication specifying the profile of physicians who comply more often with clinical practice guidelines: these are especially women, specialists, having recently completed their studies, frequently using a computer, working in groups [5], and we have also seen that in the study by Lazaro on clinical inertia in the treatment of hypercholesterolemia, physicians who often went to conventions followed guidelines better [6].

Two meta-analyses are available on the effect of physician Continuing Medical Education on their medical practices and on health indicators of patients. A Cochrane meta-analysis of studies carried out between 1999 and 2006 highlighted an improvement of about 6 % in guideline compliance and of 3 % regarding health indicators of patients treated by the physicians involved; this meta-analysis would suggest an effect of the format of meetings and their didactic nature [7]. The value of repeatedly using multimedia appears also in the analysis of the literature by Mazmanian et al. [8] One can also currently witness the advent of e-learning in teaching practitioners treatment algorithms [9, 10].

## Role of "Opinion Leaders"

Finally, it's through Continuing Medical Education that one can see the true role of "opinion leaders": by this one means a respected person whose charisma can exert an effect of changing the behavior of listeners [11]. A Cochrane meta-analysis suggests that opinion leaders can certainly influence physicians' practices, but in fact without actually being more effective than other techniques for training physicians, for example audit and feedback techniques [12, 13].

## Reminder and Feedback Systems

Phillips' diabetes team carried out a study in which residents were randomized into two groups: in the "intervention" group, residents received a "reminder" in the form of an electronic spreadsheet specifying for the patient that they are going to see the latest lab results, the treatment, and guidelines on the treatment to be given. Moreover they were subjected to a feedback method consisting of a five minute interview with an endocrinologist, every 15 days, with the purpose of analyzing their behavior, especially in relation to guidelines of the American Diabetes Association. The results of the study show that it is particularly the "feedback" part of the intervention on the improvement of practices which proved to be effective. Moreover, the effect of the "reminder" appeared to have less effect after 3 years, which appeared to be less the case for residents benefitting from the feedback method [14].

Still in the field of diabetes, it can be interesting to note a study whose results were negative. O'Connor et al. studied the effect of feedback when information was given only to the patient, only to the physician, or to both. For example, physicians received every 4 months a list of their patients with reminders of HbA1c or LDL-cholesterol measures which had not been carried out, and giving guidelines if these two parameters were not corrected without there having been treatment intensification within 4 months. The feedback consisted of every 4 months giving physicians their rank among the physicians in their environment, regarding the percentage of their patients that were controlled. Patients also received a reminder of their situation, guidelines regarding adherence and the next appointment. Yet the results were negative: patient HbA1c did not improve and even deteriorated in patients with HbA1c above 8 %. In fact the study showed that patient appointment times were, contrary to what was expected, longer. According to the authors' interpretation, these results could be due to a negative reaction from patients regarding the information letter, and, on the physician's side, to the fact that the lists of patients were sent to them every 4 months, and not before each appointment, and that the feedback information occurred too late [15].

In the field of hypertension, the study by Roumie et al. consisted of randomizing health care providers into three groups. The first group of physicians received an e-mail reminding them of one of the recent guidelines regarding the treatment of hypertension (control group); the second group of physicians in addition received a computer alert specific to each patient informing her of the three most recent blood pressure measurements and proposing a treatment modification if necessary; patients of a third group of physicians (who received guidelines and the alert) received an educational document emphasizing adherence and lifestyle changes. The results were clear: in this third group of patients, blood pressure was better controlled, while there was no difference in blood pressure levels between patients treated by the first two groups of physicians, suggesting a major impact of patient education [16]. Another publication by Roumie [17] regarding this study made it possible to analyze physicians' behavior and their barriers to treatment intensification: the results were in accordance with the model by Cabana [18] (see Chap. 4, page vv).

Incidentally, this effect of patient education emphasizes that insufficient education of patients also represents an aspect of clinical inertia (what's more, the need to include patient education in the management of patients with chronic diseases is now part of clinical practice guidelines). As noted by Moser, lack of time could well be but an alibi: it takes less than 3 min to remind someone that hypertension can be asymptomatic, that treatment is in general for life, that lifestyle changes are beneficial but that in general medications are needed, that when blood pressure is normalized one must continue treatment, finally that if one takes one's treatment properly one can avoid the complications of hypertension [19]. André Scheen et al. also suggested that the fact that the physician has integrated patient education in her practice could represent a comprehensive approach to care which could contribute to keeping her safe from clinical inertia [20].

In Germany, Lüders et al. also studied the effect of physician training on the following of guidelines in treatment of hypertension, accompanied by a feedback method giving them information on blood pressure control of each patient and indicating to them if it had improved or if they needed to intensify treatment. Physicians in a control group did not receive this intervention. There was no difference in the number of treatment modifications or the dose adjustments of medications. Nevertheless, the authors report that in the "intervention" group, there was a 6 % decrease in the rate of clinical inertia (lack of treatment modification even though blood pressure readings are elevated). In this group of patients, they observed a discrete improvement in the percentage of patients having reached the target [21].

In general, it seems that the effects of educational interventions on physician compliance with clinical practice guidelines are therefore variable and often limited; nevertheless, the quality of the level of evidence provided by these meta-analyses is limited by the heterogeneity of the studies analyzed [22]. More recently, a cluster randomized trial performed in Belgium investigated the effect of interventions including evidence-based treatment protocol, annual benchmarking, postgraduate education, case-coaching for general practitioners and patient education. Endpoints improved significantly after intervention: there was a significant decrease in HbA1c, systolic blood pressure, and LDL-cholesterol [23]. By contrast, the effect of an educational toolkit in improving quality of care or cardiovascular outcomes in a large population with diabetes in Ontario was recently investigated in a pragmatic cluster randomized trial. Despite being relatively easy and inexpensive to implement, the printed educational materials were not effective, neither on mortality or non-fatal myocardial infarction rates, which were the primary outcomes in the administrative data study, nor in the use of statin, which was the primary outcome in the clinical data study. A limitation is the high baseline rate of statin prescription in this population [24]. The difference in outcome of these last two studies highlights the effect of the choice of outcome.

## Facilitators

### Simplify Treatments, Use Treatments Having Fewer Side Effects

We have seen in the previous chapter that complexity can be the cause of indecision, since it is one of the elements which make it that a decision is *difficult*. Moreover, the number of pills to be taken is a well known cause of patient nonadherence and the physician may hesitate to prescribe "one more pill", adopting therefore behavior that falls under clinical inertia [25]: it suffices to think of the number of pills that a patient with several vascular risk factors must take. That's why simplification of treatments, using combined forms of medications can be a means not only to improve patient adherence, but also to overcome clinical inertia of health care providers [26–28].

Moreover, fear of treatment side effects (for example, fear of hypoglycemia and weight gain in the case of insulin therapy) can also be a cause of treatment refusal by the patient, and, consequently, clinical inertia on the part of the physician who hesitates at the prospect of this refusal which she is expecting. This is why one can imagine that, in diabetes treatment, the arrival of new medications in the incretin axis (GLP-1 analogues, DPP-4 inhibitors) which do not have these side effects, may also lead to a decrease in physician clinical inertia regarding poor glycemic control [29, 30].

### Overcoming Decisional Uncertainty Through Protocols

We have also seen that uncertainty regarding the decision to be made is a major cause of preference for the *status quo*. It's here that giving specific algorithms to the clinician can help her to leave her indecision which is the cause of her clinical inertia. That's the value of diagnostic decision trees which lead the practitioner by the hand in her approach, and one understands why they take on so much educational importance in medical studies.

From a therapeutic point of view, one can, as Alan Morris does, distinguish "protocols" from guidelines: an example of a protocol is that which he developed for the decision regarding insulin infusion rate in hyperglycemic patients in Intensive Care Units [31]. It was possible to analyze the reasons that oppose the use of this protocol by nurses [32]: fear of hypoglycemia, and uncertainty in particular. Regarding the chronic management of type 2 diabetes, Phillips' team showed that giving a simple algorithm of titration of treatment to physicians was accompanied by an increase in the percentage of appointments where treatment was intensified and an improvement in glycemic control of patients [33]. Gandara et al. described, in the management of hypertension, an alert system via e-mail for generalists triggered after review of the patient's electronic medical record by a nurse and a physician, but this system has not yet been assessed [34].

In the same line of thinking, uncertainty regarding the reality of elevated blood pressure readings represents, we have seen, one of the causes of clinical inertia. A study showed that using an automated blood pressure measurement device reduced clinical inertia, but the value of this study is limited due to lack of control group [35]. Recently, a cluster randomized trial, comparing centers having a means of overcoming uncertainty (physicians in the "intervention" group received a graph representing previous blood pressure readings) showed a positive effect on treatment intensification and, significantly, on blood pressure readings in this study lasting over three years [36].

## Organizational Aspects

### Electronic Reminders and Electronic Medical Record

Use by physicians of an Electronic Medical Record can help them, in part through the use of electronic reminders and facilitated exchanges with patients, to implement certain elements of monitoring, even incite them to prescribe certain treatments [37, 38]. For example, an American study, lasting three years, including 46 health care centers randomized by cluster and regarding 27,207 diabetic patients, clearly showed the advantage of Electronic Medical Records over paper records [39]: a positive effect was observed on the carrying out of care standards (receipt of HbA1c result, prescription of microalbuminuria measure, of a dilated eye examination, prescription of angiotensin-converting-enzyme inhibitors or angiotensin receptor blockers, of pneumococcal vaccination) and on intermediate criteria: HbA1c, LDL-cholesterol, blood pressure, Body Mass Index, nonsmoker status.

In another study, the value of exchanges via e-mail over two months between physicians and patients was demonstrated in a study of 35,423 diabetic and/or hypertensive patients, covered by the Californian health insurance program Kaiser Permanente: an improvement in certain quality criteria and biological parameters was also observed [40]. We will see later how patients, by getting involved in their treatment, can improve the quality of care which is given to them.

## Disease Management

One can start from a comment by Perlin and Pogach in their analysis of the causes of clinical inertia [41]. The importance of organizational aspects can be demonstrated in the analysis of different centers involved in the Veteran Health Administration: there is more variability in management practices of diabetic patients between centers depending on the administration than between individual physicians [42]: what makes the difference between these centers, is the organization of frequent feedback on quality indicators, designation of a "guideline champion", and to think that guidelines are applicable in common practice [43].

"Disease Management" therefore has the goal of improving the quality of chronic disease management through organizational measures. An example in France is the implementation of the patient support program called Sophia, in which the Public Health Insurance System, while informing their physicians, offers diabetic patients educational documents and the opportunity to have a telephone interview with a nurse. Preliminary assessment results seem positive, showing a significantly greater (but small) increase, between 2008 and 2009, in all monitoring indicators (ophthalmology appointment, electrocardiogram, dental appointment, frequency of HbA1c measure, measurement of LDL-cholesterol, measurement of proteinuria/microalbuminuria, measurement of serum creatinine) in members of the Sophia program [44].

It is essential that this type of program be carried out in collaboration with the attending physician so that she does not feel stripped of her responsibility in the quality of care: Disease Management programs must help physicians in an educational way to progress in overcoming clinical inertia and should not give the impression that one can improve the quality of care despite their clinical inertia, as if they were, in the end, "beyond help" [45].

## The Coordinated Health Care Plan

One can quote here the contribution of the French law of 2004, which invites everyone having right to the Public Health Insurance System to register in a Coordinated Health Care Plan, organized by the attending physician: According to Michel Varroud-Vial, the very existence of this system, by giving the general practitioner the responsibility of organizing it, may represent a means of overcoming clinical inertia [46]. Within this framework, a synergy between the attending physician and the specialist who have different positions in the management of chronic diseases, especially in diabetology, could be beneficial [47].

## The Problem of Time and Telemedicine

There is no denying it: lack of time is an underlying cause of clinical inertia. It's because the physician lacks the time that she puts off till tomorrow actions that she can judge as not being a priority, faced with more urgent "competing demands" of her patient, and we have seen many examples. We have also seen through Anderson in his review on *The psychology of doing nothing* [48] that it is when it lacks the time that the human mind finds that a decision is "difficult", the consequence being refuge in the *status quo*. Finding facilitators to overcome the lack of time is an essential investigative axis to overcome clinical inertia. One must tackle the medical shortages but also perhaps find other systems to promote medical activities other than fee-for-service, in order to encourage physicians to consecrate appointments dedicated to the management of long-term treatment of chronic diseases, that is to say to their essentially silent aspect, which they alone are able to appreciate. Incidentally, this passes also through a true promotion of patient education, whose requirement in the management of chronic diseases is now inscribed in the French law on Hospitals, Patients, Health and Territories (loi *Hôpital, Patients, Santé, Territoires* – HPST).

Another means to overcome physicians' lack of time is based on the use of telemedicine [49], also inscribed in the HPST law. For example, the fact that the dilated eye examination in diabetes is insufficiently performed, due to lack of ophthalmologists, can be resolved by the use of retinal photography with remote analysis of photographs of the ocular fundus [50]; by decreasing the difficulty of obtaining the examination, this can contribute to improve its prescription. One can also evoke analysis of a treatment diary by remote computer [51] or see in the establishment of an interprofessionalism, which consists of delegating to nurses certain medical tasks, a solution to the problem of clinical inertia, if it appears that physician lack of time is responsible.

It is interesting to note that in our work devoted to patient nonadherence regarding her treatment [52], the relationship to temporality also emerged as central on two levels: it takes time, on a day-to-day basis, to treat oneself and one must be able to project oneself into the future to understand the sense of taking care of oneself. The same is true of overcoming clinical inertia: the physician must have *the time to treat* and she must give, we will see, priority to the future of her patient. The relationship to temporality is clearly the common node in the double issue of nonadherence and clinical inertia.

## Reinforcement

Can the physician reinforce her desire to implement clinical practice guidelines? We will consider successively the incentives which can come from public authorities, from her patients, what she can expect from others, and finally the possibility of self-commitment.

### Incentive by Public Authorities: Pay for Performance

Thus, the existence of clinical practice guidelines is not sufficient to avoid clinical inertia, although this is in fact their purpose. Should incentives be envisaged, such as financial bonuses for performance ("Pay for Performance", often called P4P), practitioners receiving a bonus based on good results?

In 2005, an initial assessment took place in the United States, showing effectiveness in improvement of certain practices (for example the screening for cervical cancer) [53]. In 2007, a study in the United States showed that Hospitals which associated a Pay for Performance policy with a "Public Reporting" initiative (publication of indicator results on a website) improved more their performance than those only subjected to the principle of Public Reporting [54]. Since, several countries have adopted a policy of Pay for Performance to incite physicians to improve their practices. Interestingly enough, use of financial incentives has also been proposed as a means to motivate individuals to adopt health behaviors, both short-term (for example acceptance of a vaccination), but also for long-term health programs (such as quitting smoking or weight loss): it has been shown that they can be effective in certain conditions [55].

Of course, several subjects of concern were quickly expressed faced with this practice, which we can summarize thus [56–60]: (1) Physicians, focusing on quantitative quality indicators, can lose an overall view of the patient (just as students only study what might be on the test!) (2) There is a risk of sterilizing innovation, due to the tendency to reward conformism; (3) This policy is expensive, and the expenditure could be put to better use; (4) There is the risk of avoiding treating difficult patients, which in fact would end up reinforcing the disparities, to the detriment of the most vulnerable patients. (5) One must emphasize the difficulty of selecting quality indicators, and one evokes "Goodhart's law": when a measurement becomes a target, it ceases to be a good measurement. (6) The choice of indicators is difficult, what one measures must be able to improve in the short-term; one is therefore forced to take intermediate markers. The target value retained as a gage of success must take into account the current uncertainty regarding the optimum level, for example due to "J-curves" which have been noted for diabetes and hypertension. It is therefore better to focus on what physicians have done; but how, then, can one distinguish clinical inertia from appropriate inaction? (7) If one pays "good doctors" more, should one pay "bad doctors" less? (8) What, ultimately, is the policy which underlies Pay for Performance: improve the quality of care or decrease health care expenditure?

This is to say that assessment of these practices is indispensable. We have several meta-analyses, carried out starting in 2010. The review by Van Herck concludes that of course, one can but expect in a field touching upon public health – "there is no magic bullets in this arena" – a heterogeneity of effects, but as a whole the consequences are often positive, rarely negative [61]. Another literature review devoted to P4P within Disease Management programs insists upon the difficulty of drawing general conclusions; only five studies assessing the impact on quality of care were identified, mostly positive, but none assessed the impact on health care expenditure [62]. A Cochrane meta-analysis of 7 randomized controlled trials provides the same conclusion: "the evidence" is not of very high quality, and though six out of 7 studies seem to indicate a positive effect on certain indicators, the authors conclude that based on available Evidence one can neither support, nor not support the Pay for Performance system [63]. The same conclusion on the variability of the effect of implementing P4P can be drawn from two recent meta-analyses [64, 65].

In France, a new agreement, signed on July 26, 2011, sanctions the generalization of Pay for Performance for general practitioners [66]: "though fee-for-service remains the foundation of physician remuneration, this agreement marks a progression towards a mixed mode of remuneration comprised of three pillars: the service, the flat rate and a remuneration for performance based on public health objectives." The system thus generalizes a measure from 2009, the "CAPI" (*Contrats d'Amélioration des Pratiques Individuelles*). In April 2011, 16,000 physicians had signed a CAPI with their Health Insurance fund, or more than 1 eligible physician out of 3. By the end of June 2010, over 70 % of signatory physicians had received a bonus at the end of the first year of implementation of the contract. With an average of 3,000 €, the bonus varied between physicians, from 1,500 € for the 10 % the least remunerated to close to 4,900 € for the 10 % the most remunerated, with a maximum amount reached of more than 17,000 €. Modest, but significant effects on the "performance" of physicians were highlighted [67]. The new agreement signed in July 2011 should allow physicians to receive up to 9,100 euros in bonus if they reach all their objectives, or a maximum "remuneration per patient of 11.4 euros" for a patient list of 800 patients.

In practice, 29 objectives are defined whose fulfillment is accounted for in 1,300 points: prevention objectives (250 points for vaccination, screening for cancers, etc.), monitoring of chronic diseases (250 points for diabetes and hypertension), mastery of expenditure objectives (400 points for prescriptions), but also management of a medical office objectives (400 points): simply keeping electronic medical records or having a prescription assistance software is attributed points (we have seen the value of the computerization of medical activities). Remuneration takes into account both the reaching of objectives as well as the progress made. A starting point, an intermediate target and an objective target, are defined for each indicator, common to all physicians.

## Incentive by Patients

In the field of hypertension, a study showed that when patients were given information documents on the treatment of hypertension and the value of adding thiazide diuretics and asking them to talk about it with their physician, the physician less often adopted the attitude consisting of putting off treatment intensification till the next appointment [68]. Likewise, the performance of home blood pressure monitoring by the patient can represent a means to decrease physician clinical inertia, as demonstrated by the meta-analysis by Agarwal [69]. Grant et al. carried out a controlled study in which patients, having access to their electronic medical record via the internet, could create a treatment program (for example indicating their wish to improve their glycemia, their blood pressure readings) which they gave to their physician. The physician intensified treatment in 51 % of cases compared to 15 % in patients in the control arm (p < 0.001) [70].

Finally, more and more people search for information on health or medicine on the internet, and a meta-analysis of 75 randomized trials showed a positive effect of information disseminated via the internet [71]. One can thus imagine that patients, informed by what they might have heard or read (the internet) moreover, help physicians to avoid clinical inertia. A randomized trial is underway to try to prove the value of this concept [72]. One can also note that initiatives such as Sophia, discussed above, have the effect of giving patients information which allows them to discuss their therapeutic project with their physician.

This is in line with what one calls patient empowerment. This is, what's more, one of the most important roles of patient education: to show her how she can become actively involved in her treatment in partnership with the health care team. It is in this sense that patient education represents, for the physician who practices it, a means of overcoming her own clinical inertia, as we have already mentioned.

## Incentive by Others: Peers, Pharmacists and Nurses

Participation in discussion groups for medical records, whether they be made up of hospital staff members or "groups of peers", like those developed in the *Société Française de Médecine Générale* [73], could represent an effective means of overcoming clinical inertia, which, it has already been said, could be a consequence of a solitary practice of medicine.

Another approach aiming to correct the effect of bias and "competing demands" which are, we have seen, causes of clinical inertia, consists of organizing an appointment with another physician, aiming specifically to take care of prevention problems. In patients with diabetes, hypertension and hypercholesterolemia, Fiscella et al. showed that this approach brought about improvement of blood pressure readings, but not of HbA1c or hypercholesterolemia. During the appointment with the peer, treatments were intensified more than in an ordinary appointment which served as a control group [74].

A study in the Netherlands, having the objective of specifying the factors associated with clinical inertia in the treatment of hypertension in diabetic patients, showed that clinical inertia was less frequent when physicians were assisted by a nurse. In the Netherlands, nurses do not have the right to make medical prescriptions, and this effect is therefore undoubtedly due to the fact that they gave advice [75].

The role of pharmacists was evoked to help the physician to avoid clinical inertia [76], but this effect is still to be proven. A study in the United States, in which pharmacists, having access to the patient's electronic record, sent a letter to the attending physicians, had little effect on the quality indicators assessed [77]. However, Carter et al. showed that collaboration between physician and pharmacist allowed a decrease in clinical inertia score and brought about improvement in blood pressure readings [78].

## Physician Self-Incentive: An Explanation Through Philosophy of Mind

One means of overcoming weakness of will is by committing oneself to act. Jon Elster recalls that Ulysses, feeling that he might succumb to temptation, knowing that his rationality is imperfect, commits himself by asking his seamen to bind him to his mast [79]. One can use this principle of precommitment as a means to avoid clinical inertia from being repeated from appointment to appointment: one commits to act "the next time" for example by telling the patient what one will do if necessary (if your glycated hemoglobin is still above 7 %, I really think that we should start insulin therapy), by writing it in the patient's record, or by writing it to a physician correspondent (in a letter given to the patient...).

Gollwitzer [80] described all the obstacles to the reaching of a goal that one has set: first one can not get going: either that, simply, one forgets that one had set the goal (because one had something else to do – let us think of "competing demands" as a cause of clinical inertia!), or that one does not seize an opportunity to take action, or that one has, at the moment of taking action, a reason to not do so. But then, one can not reach one's goal because along one's way, one succumbed to other temptations, to a bad mood, etc. A means of overcoming these obstacles is to call upon what he calls an "implementation intention". This is an intention which has a form of "if – then": if I am in situation X, then I will implement behavior Y which will allow me to reach goal Z. In fact, this is not a matter of specifying *what* I want, but of stating the *when, where, and how* of what I will do to achieve what I want. One can find in Gollwitzer's article data suggesting that this strategy is more effective in leading to the carrying out of one's goal.

It appears to us that the strategy which consists of deciding to avoid clinical inertia by committing to intensify treatment at the next appointment comes back precisely to forming an "implementation intention". One can also liken this strategy to another philosophical concept, described by the philosopher Richard Holton, that of resolution [81]: this is a special form of intention whose characteristic is precisely to be able to overcome inclinations, contrary to a project, which could manifest themselves: if a new desire proves to be stronger than a usual intention and if the subject changes her mind, one would say simply that she is fickle; if this new desire wins over a resolution, one would say that she demonstrates weakness of will. Yet certain persons are able to stay the course that they have set themselves. They succeed because they have a special capacity which allows them to mentally repeat to themselves what it is they have committed to – since one has to do so if one wants to prevail – but without this mental repetition leading to a reconsideration of their decision. This is what *willpower* does. Is willpower applicable to overcoming clinical inertia? Is this not the principle of the process of "assessment of professional practices" or the search for "quality" which are implemented in many professional contexts, including the context of care?

## Force of Habit

Finally, is this implementation intention not analogous to what the philosopher John Searle called "prior intention"? To adopt the vocabulary of *Intentionality* by Searle [82], which we have already mentioned (see page 74) – an attitude is "intentional" if it has a content, for example, I believe *it is raining*: "it is raining" is the content of my belief. But the fact that it is *truly* raining is the condition of satisfaction of my belief. In the intention "I have the intention *to apply this guideline*", the fact that I actually apply this guideline is the condition of satisfaction of my attitude, here, the fact of having an intention, which Searle calls "intention in action". But this "intention in action" is in turn the condition of satisfaction of another more general intention, which he calls prior intention, for example "I have the intention of improving my practice". According to Searle, the prior intention causes the intention in action.

This hypothesis could explain *the force of habit*. We have proposed that its mechanism is to avoid having to call upon a prior intention [83]: I've gotten into the habit of taking the stairs; at the start the intention to do so was caused by the prior intention to lose weight etc.; involving prior intention brought about a feeling of effort, that which one feels when one exerts one's *volition*, which is this action which makes it that one enables oneself to act, as the philosopher Joëlle Proust states [84]; but since the action has become a habit, I do it without thinking about it: I do it, and that's it. We have proposed that this could explain certain behaviors of patient adherence: the patient has gotten into the habit of taking her pills [83]. We can now attempt to apply the same mechanism to the prevention of clinical inertia: the physician *has gotten into the habit* of prescribing a dilated eye examination each year to all diabetic patients; *she does so apparently without effort*.

The preceding discussion shows again the homology between patient nonadherence and physician clinical inertia (phenomena are homologous, and not only analogous, if they have a common mechanism) [85]. The use of philosophical explanations of these two phenomena should not be surprising: in this book, we have tried to answer the question "how is clinical inertia possible?" Yet, as we have put forth in the introduction of this book, to ask how something is *possible* typically represents the task of the philosopher [86, 87].

## Can One Avoid Cognitive Biases?

As emphasized by Croskerry, to reflect on the way that we think and feel about our emotions represents a "cognitive imperative" for the physician [88], and he insists upon the need to teach future physicians the foundations of medical reason emphasizing the different "heuristics" which, as mental short-cuts, are clearly useful in diagnosis (we think in particular of the representativeness heuristic) but are often a source of bias. The experienced clinician is one who, perhaps unconsciously, has learned, undoubtedly at times at her own expense, to distrust her own reasoning.

Epstein et al. described the role of this ability of psychological self-monitoring which consists for the physician "of seeking, integrating, and responding to both external and internal data about one's own performance" [89]. This capacity requires several elements: motivation, attention, curiosity, and certain mental habits which are the capacity to view information anew, to doubt, to tell oneself that the first diagnosis is not the right one, in brief to ask: is this diagnosis the only one possible? Teaching young physicians to cultivate this state of mind could perhaps subsequently, to a certain extent, keep them safe from clinical inertia.

One could think that clinical practice guidelines are there to help us avoid making errors resulting from the bias introduced through the use of heuristics, and some have even pleaded for the education of physicians and future physicians in Bayesian principles of reasoning. Of course, above we have given many examples showing that application of protocols could help physicians or nurses to decide in a context of uncertainty. Nevertheless, this is definitely to forget that our reasoning cannot do without heuristics. Undoubtedly, it is better to recognize their existence and try to overcome their potential unfortunate effect: thus, as Bradley states, "At the bedside, asking yourself whether your initial diagnosis is the only possibility or whether there could be something you are missing is a cognitive forcing strategy that is not too time consuming or taxing and yet could yield benefits." [90] The same principle could be applied when the physician *renews a prescription*.

Phillips, in his initial publication [91], stated that one of the causes of clinical inertia was denial. This is exerted in fact on two levels: on the one hand, we have seen, by negation of the gravity of the situation (underestimation of blood pressure readings, cholesterol level etc.), on the other hand by negation of the existence of the clinical inertia phenomenon itself regarding one's own practice. Here one can cite the study by Wexler et al. [92] which showed regarding treatment of hypertension, conducted on 28 physicians, that they "strongly agreed" (n=3) or "agreed" (n=25) with the statement: "I do a good job of treating my patients' hypertension" and (n=26/28) that the primary problem was patient nonadherence. Twenty-seven physicians claimed to be familiar with the JNC 7 Guideline (The seventh Report of the Joint National Committee on the Evaluation, Detection, and Treatment of Hypertension). Nevertheless, the *median* value they gave for thresholds to intensify treatment was 140/90, which means that only one in two physicians declared intensify treatment if blood pressure was above 140/90.

## Emotional Reversal: Using Emotions to Overcome Clinical Inertia

In the previous chapter, we have demonstrated how emotions can intervene in clinical inertia, and among them, we have cited fear and regret (what Feinstein calls chagrin) [93]: it's because she is afraid of a hemorrhagic stroke, and that she does not wish to regret it that the physician does not prescribe anticoagulant treatment in a patient however at high risk of embolic stroke. These two emotions belong typically to what one calls, in the taxonomy of emotions, negative emotions.

Fear, in the physician's mind, can also have an effect of avoidance of clinical inertia, which is to avoid being blamed for not having followed a guideline: this is in fact the feeling of shame (another negative emotion – does the method of Public Reporting not call upon this emotion here?). She may be also afraid of a lawsuit: in fact often this fear here leads to another type of lack of following of guidelines, which consists of prescribing too many lab tests, contrary to that required by guidelines, this is therefore typically what one calls "defensive medicine" [94].

## Concern: The Philosophical Dimension of Care

Another emotion which can allow one to avoid clinical inertia is concern. In our work on patient adherence [52] we recall that, in English, the word *care* is used to define both the concept of medical care (for example the journal *Diabetes Care* focuses on diabetes treatment) and concern. In fact, as demonstrated by the American philosopher Harry Frankfurt outside any medical context in his book *The Importance of What We Care About*, there is a relationship between what one is concerned about – *what we care about* – and what is *important* to us [95]. But he also showed that when we consider that something is important for us, we place ourselves in a reflection about our future: I may desire to eat some vanilla ice-cream, but it's not very important to me. If something actually is important to me, if I care about it, it is that it has a dimension which concerns the future.

We have thus proposed [52] that one solution to clinical inertia is the use of a form of concern that could be described as fear of what can occur to the patient, *in the future*. The philosopher Stephen Darwall [96] uses the example of someone who encounters a person who has lost her son: she can demonstrate empathy and imagine the terrible feelings which this person experiences. But after all, she could be indifferent to this, she could even rejoice with sadism. Darwall calls sympathy the *emotion* which consists of experiencing the feeling that a person is in distress and that this distress asks to be relieved. But beware: in the case in point, if the physician is only interested in the *present* distress of the patient to whom she offers insulin, only in her fear, and if she has the intention to relieve this distress, she will not prescribe insulin and will demonstrate clinical inertia. We have therefore proposed that the emotion which could prevent the physician from falling into the trap of clinical inertia is to demonstrate sympathy, as Darwall states, but in defining sympathy as the emotion triggered by the thought of *future* risks which threaten the patient which she treats [52].

## Implementing Positive Emotions: Emotional Reversal

Negative emotions have their equivalent, positive emotions. One can adopt the taxonomy of emotions proposed by Elster [97]: thus, sadness and fear, on the one side, and joy and hope, on the other, are negative and positive emotions caused by bad or good things which have happened or which can happen; disappointment and regret, on the one side, and relief, on the other, are negative and positive emotions which are caused by good or bad things which could have happened, but did not happen. To the negative emotions which are shame, hatred, anger, disgust, respond positive emotions which are pride, love, admiration, appeal. For Spinoza, fear is pain, the same can be said for regret. Yet we wish to avoid pain: "[…] All the endeavors of a man affected by pain are directed to removing that pain […] A man affected by pleasure has no desire further than to preserve it." (*The Ethics*, IV. *On human bondage*, Proposition 37).

We propose to call "emotional reversal" the fact of trying, deliberately, to use positive emotions in care. Rather than pain, pleasure, than fear, hope, than regret, relief, and, particularly, rather than shame, pride. Indeed, Spinoza states again: "Desire arising from pleasure is, other conditions being equal, stronger than desire arising from pain." (*The Ethics*, IV, Proposition 18).

## Physician Optimism and Pessimism

Perhaps this use of positive emotions comes back simply to a demonstration of *optimism*. Optimism has essentially been considered from the point of view of the person herself: an optimistic person is one which, in general, considers positively *her own* future, and numerous studies show that optimism intervenes favorably in health behaviors, as shown in the recent review by Carver devoted to this character trait [98]; one can therefore ask if being more or less optimistic intervenes in the way in which the physician takes into account the future *of her patient*: if one recalls the Regulatory Focus Theory by Higgins [99], whose relevance, we have seen, Veazie and Qian [100] have shown that for interpreting the clinical inertia phenomenon, the fact of favoring a promotion focus over a prevention focus, which, according to the authors, keeps her safe from clinical inertia, could be related to this character trait of the physician.

Can one, then, become optimistic if one is of a pessimistic nature? The answers that Carver gives to this question at the end of his review [98] could be relevant to our issue: in particular, it is a matter of overcoming a pessimism which would be unjustified, to recognize that pessimism is often linked to the disproportionate nature of what one is not able to reach, to know therefore to seek realistic objectives, but also to guard against ill founded optimism.

## Trust, Pride and Self-Approval

Finally we wish to show how one can, based on the notion of trust in care, arrive at the notion of pride and self-approval, two positive emotions which, *when they are anticipated*, could represent a powerful driving force to overcome clinical inertia.

How do patients accept "one more pill"? A recent study, in which 64 % of patients agreed to intensify treatment, gave as independent factors significantly explaining their acceptance of the new medication the following elements: negatively was the risk of side effects of the medication (RR 0.49) and adherence problems to other medications (RR 0.72), but, positively was the feeling that health depends on medications (RR 1.50), and finally, *trust in their physician* (RR 1.30). On the contrary, control of blood pressure and the number of medications did not intervene significantly [101]. Inversely, a study highlighted a significant effect of trust on adherence to drug-taking in treatment of inflammatory bowel diseases [102].

Among the factors which determine the trust that the patient has in her physician, one finds appreciation of skills (care placed in assessment of the situation and the quality of treatments prescribed), but also the capacity to understand the uniqueness of the patient's experience, the clarity of communication, the capacity to construct a true partnership and to demonstrate respect [103]. A study tried to rank the importance of determinants of trust [104]. One finds here the importance of the quality of communication, in its two aspects, verbal and nonverbal. A recent meta-analysis confirmed the essential role of communication in patient adherence: the risk of nonadherence is increased by 19 % in patients whose physician has poor communication capacities [105].

We note in fact that all practice of medicine involves a relationship of trust: to answer questions, lend oneself to a clinical examination, accept the treatment. Yet, philosopher Gloria Origgi states [106], one trusts someone if one assumes that she has an interest in being worthy of it: trust creates the existence of reciprocal, or "encapsulated" [107], interests. She adds that the person in whom someone trusts will have the tendency to be worthy of it since, she suggests, human beings love to find themselves under the approving gaze of others. One can propose, by transposing this analysis of trust to the subject which concerns us, that trust appears thus in the end not only as an essential driving force of patient adherence, *but also, for the physician, as protection against clinical inertia* – the physician asking herself the question: am I worthy of her trust?

We propose therefore that the physician, anticipating the pride – a positive emotion – that she might feel at the thought of being worthy of the patient's trust, can, through this, keep herself safe from clinical inertia. To find oneself under the approving gaze of others, is this not perhaps one of the meanings of the end of the Hippocratic Oath: "If I keep this oath faithfully, may I [be] respected by all humanity and in all times; but if I transgress or violate it, may the reverse be my lot"? Undoubtedly one must add that the physician should also have at heart to avoid clinical inertia if she wants to find herself under her own approving gaze. We have proposed that self-approval – again a positive emotion – is a condition of care on the part of the patient [52]. It could, on the part of the physician, be the condition of avoidance of clinical inertia, when it risks being the consequence of choices made by the emotional part of medical reason: this would be the victory of self-approval, the highest emotion there is according to Spinoza [108], above other emotions.

Finally, concern, which, we have seen, defines care can also be seen in this emotional reversal: Spinoza stated that hope is an inconstant pleasure arising from the idea of something past or future, whereof we to a certain extent doubt the issue, and that fear is an inconstant pain arising from the idea of something past or future whereof we to a certain extent doubt the issue; he stated that from these definitions it follows that there is no hope unmingled with fear, and no fear unmingled with hope [109].

It appears to us then that concern, *which is care*, is this emotion that the physician feels when she is *both* in hope and fear, because she finds herself in a situation of uncertainty faced with the risk to which the patient is exposing: the uncertainty which governs the whole issue of clinical inertia. Schrödinger's cat is still *both* living and dead, and Einstein's boxes are still closed. Faced with this indetermination, one has to, in the end, make a bet. This bet, the physician must make while letting herself be guided by her medical reason: it alone can help her to decide, between the *status quo* and a change of treatment, what will best protect the future of her patient.

# References

1. Schiff GD, Galanter WL, Duhig J, Lodolce AE, Koronkowski MJ, Lambert BL. Principles of conservative prescribing. Arch Intern Med. 2011;17:1433–40.
2. Wegwarth O, Gaissmaier W, Gigerenzer G. Smart strategies for doctors and doctors-in-training: heuristics in medicine. Med Educ. 2009;43:721–8.
3. Reach G. Patient nonadherence and healthcare-provider inertia are clinical myopia. Diabetes Metab. 2008;34:382–5.
4. Reach G. Non-observance et inertie clinique: deux mises en défaut de la relation de soin. In: Manuel de Médecine, Santé et Sciences Humaines, Collège des Enseignants de Sciences Humaines et Sociales en Médecine et Santé. Paris: Les Belles Lettres; 2011, p 284–92.
5. Sammer CE, Lykens K, Singh KP. Physician characteristics and the reported effect of evidence-based practice guidelines. Health Serv Res. 2008;43:569–81.
6. Lazaro P, Murga N, Aguilar D, Hernandez-Presa MA. Therapeutic Inertia in the outpatient management of dyslipidemia in patients with ischemic heart disease. The Inertia Study. Rev Esp Cardiol. 2010;63:1428–37.
7. Forsetlund L, Bjorndal A, Rashidian A, Jamtvedt G, O'Brien MA, Wolf F, Davis D, Odgaard-Jensen J, Oxman AD. Continuing education meetings and workshops: effects on professional practice and health care outcomes. Cochrane Database Syst Rev. 2009;(2):CD003030.
8. Mazmanian PE, Davis DA, Galbraith R. Continuing Medical Education effect on clinical outcomes. Chest. 2009;135:49S–55.
9. Cook CB, Wilson RD, Hovan MJ, Hull BP, Gray RJ, Apsey HA. Development of computer-based training to enhance resident physician management of inpatient diabetes. J Diabetes Sci Technol. 2009;3:1377–87.
10. Sperl-Hillen JM, O'Connor PJ, Rush WA, Johnson PE, Gilmer T, Biltz G, Asche SE, Ekstrom HL. Simulated physician learning program improves glucose control in adults with diabetes. Diabetes Care. 2010;33:1727–33.
11. Carpenter CR, Sherbino J. How does an "opinion leader" change my practice ? CJEM. 2010;12:431–4.
12. Flodgren G, Parmelli E, Doumit G, Gattellari M, O'Brien MA, Grimshaw J, Eccles MP. Local opinion leaders: effects on professional practice and health care outcomes. Cochrane Database Syst Rev. 2011;(8):CD000125.
13. Jamtvedt G, Young JM, Kristoffersen DT, Thomson O'Brien MA, Oxman AD. Audit and feedback: effects on professional practice and health care outcomes. Cochrane Database Syst Rev. 2006;(2). doi: 10.1002/14651858.CD000259.
14. Ziemer DC, Doyle JP, Barnes CS, Branch Jr WT, Cook CB, El-Kebbi IM, Gallina DL, Kolm P, Rhee MK, Phillips LS. An intervention to overcome clinical inertia and improve diabetes mellitus control in a primary care setting: Improving Primary Care of African Americans with Diabetes (IPCAAD) 8. Arch Intern Med. 2006;166:507–13.
15. O'Connor PJ, Sperl-Hillen J, Johnson PE, Rush WA, Crain AL. Customized feedback to patients and providers failed to improve safety or quality of diabetes care: a randomized trial. Diabetes Care. 2009;32:1158–63.
16. Roumie CL, Elasy TA, Greevy R, Griffin MR, Liu X, Stone WJ, Wallston KA, Dittus RS, Alvarez V, Cobb J, Speroff T. Improving blood pressure control through provider education, provider alerts, and patient education: a cluster randomized trial. Ann Intern Med. 2006;145:165–75.
17. Roumie CL, Elasy TA, Wallston KA, Pratt S, Greevy RA, Liu X, Alvarez V, Dittus RS, Speroff T. Clinical inertia: a common barrier to changing provider prescribing behavior. Jt Comm J Qual Patient Saf. 2007;33:277–85.
18. Cabana MD, Rand CS, Powe NR, Wu AW, Wilson MH, Abboud P-AC, Rubin HR. Why don't physicians follow clinical practice guidelines? A framework for improvement. JAMA. 1999;282:1458–67.

19. Moser M. Physician or clinical inertia: what it is? Is it realy a problem? And what can be done about it? J Clin Hypertens. 2009;11:1–4.
20. Scheen AJ, Bourguignon JP, Guillaume M, et les membres du Programme EUDORA. L'Éducation Thérapeutique: une solution pour vaincre l'inertie clinique et le défaut d'observance. Rev Med Liège. 2010;65:250–5.
21. Lüders S, Schrader J, Schmieder RE, Smolka W, Wegscheider K, Bestehorn K. Improvement of hypertension management by structured physician education and feedback system: cluster randomized trial. Eur J Cardiovasc Prev Rehabil. 2010;17:271–9.
22. Boaz A, Baeza J, Fraser A. Effective implementation of research into practice: an overview of systematic reviews of the health literature. BMC Research Notes. 2011;4:212. http://www.biomedcentral.com/1756-0500/4/212. Accessed 21 Apr 2014.
23. Goderis G, Borgermans L, Grol R, Van Den Broeke C, Boland B, Verbeke G, Carbonez A, Mathieu C, Heyrman J. Start improving the quality of care for people with type 2 diabetes through a general practice support program: a cluster randomized trial. Diabetes Res Clin Pract. 2010;88:56–64.
24. Shah BR, Bhattacharyya O, Yu CH, Mamdani MM, Parsons JA, Straus SE, Zwarenstein M. Effect of an educational toolkit on quality of care: a pragmatic cluster randomized trial. PLoS Med. 2014;11(2):e1001588. doi:10.1371/journal.pmed.1001588.
25. Bailey CJ, Kodack M. Patient adherence to medication requirements for therapy of type 2 diabetes. Int J Clin Pract. 2011;65:314–22.
26. Basile J, Neutel J. Overcoming clinical inertia to achieve blood pressure goals: the role of fixed-dose combination therapy. Ther Adv Cardiovasc Dis. 2010;4:119–27.
27. Scheen AJ, Lefèbvre PJ, Kulbertus H. Prévention cardio-vasculaire: la "polypill", une solution pour vaincre l'inertie clinique et le manque d'observance? Rev Med Liege. 2010;65:267–72.
28. Chrysant SG. Single-pill triple-combination therapy: an alternative to multiple-drug treatment of hypertension. Postgrad Med. 2011;123:21–31.
29. Nicolucci A, Rossi MC. Incretin-based therapies: a new potential treatment approach to overcome clinical inertia in type 2 diabetes. Acta Biomed. 2008;79:184–91.
30. Triplitt C. Improving treatment success rates for type 2 diabetes: recommendations for a changing environment. Am J Manag Care. 2010;16:S195–200.
31. Morris AH, Orme Jr J, Truwit JD, Steingrub J, Grissom C, Lee KH, Li GL, Thompson BT, Brower R, Tidswell M, Bernard GR, Sorenson D, Sward K, Zheng H, Schoenfeld D, Warner H. A replicable method for blood glucose control in critically Ill patients. Crit Care Med. 2008;36:1787–95.
32. Sward K, Orme Jr J, Sorenson D, Baumann L, Morris AH, Reengineering Critical Care Clinical Research Investigators. Reasons for declining computerized insulin protocol recommendations: application of a framework. J Biomed Inform. 2008;41:488–97.
33. Miller CD, Ziemer DC, Kolm P, El-Kebbi IM, Cook CB, Gallina DL, Doyle JP, Barnes CS, Phillips LS. Use of a glucose algorithm to direct diabetes therapy improves A1C outcomes and defines an approach to assess provider behavior. Diabetes Educ. 2006;32:533–45.
34. Gandara E, Moniz TT, Dolan ML, Melia C, Dudley J, Smith A, Kachalia A. Improving adherence to treatment guidelines: a blueprint. Crit Pathw Cardiol. 2009;8:139–45.
35. Kiberd J, Panek R, Kiberd B. Strategies to reduce clinical inertia in hypertensive kidney transplant recipients. BMC Nephrol. 2007;8:10. doi:10.1186/1471-2369-8-10.
36. Hyman DJ, Pavlik VN, Greisinger AJ, Chan W, Bayona J, Mansyur C, Simms V, Pool J. Effect of a physician uncertainty reduction intervention on blood pressure in uncontrolled hypertensives-A Cluster Randomized Trial. J Gen Intern Med. 2012;27:413–9. PMID: 22033742.
37. Varroud-Vial M. Improving diabetes management with electronic medical records. Diabetes Metab. 2011;37:S48–52.
38. Benhamou PY. Improving diabetes management with electronic health records and patients' health records. Diabetes Metab. 2011;37:S53–6.
39. Cebul RD, Love TE, Jain AK, Hebert CJ. Electronic health records and quality of diabetes care. N Engl J Med. 2011;365:825–33.

40. Zhou YY, Kanter MH, Wang JJ, Garrido T. Improved quality at Kaiser Permanente through e-mail between physicians and patients. Health Aff. 2010;29:1370–5.
41. Perlin JB, Pogach LM. Improving the outcomes of metabolic conditions: managing momentum to overcome clinical inertia. Ann Int Med. 2006;144:525–7.
42. Krein SL, Hofer TP, Kerr EA, Hayward RA. Whom should we profile? Examining diabetes care practice variation among primary care providers, provider groups, and health care facilities. Health Serv Res. 2002;37:1159–80.
43. Ward MM, Yankey JW, Vaughn TE, BootsMiller BJ, Flach SD, Welke KF, Pendergast JF, Perlin J, Doebbeling BN. Physician process and patient outcome measures for diabetes care: relationships to organizational characteristics. Med Care. 2004;42:840–50.
44. Sophia, le service d'accompagnement de l'Assurance Maladie pour les personnes atteintes de maladie chronique. http://www.ameli.fr/fileadmin/user_upload/documents/DP_sophia_220108.pdf. Accessed 21 Apr 2014.
45. Reach G. Le malade, son médecin, et le "disease manager". Médecine des Maladies Métaboliques. 2007;1:83–7.
46. Varroud-Vial M. Le parcours de soin: une solution ou une contrainte supplémentaire? Médecine des Maladies Métaboliques. 2011;5 Suppl 2:S81–5.
47. Avignon A, Attali C, Sultan A, Ferrat E, Le Breton J. Clinical inertia: viewpoints of general practitioners and diabetologists. Diabetes Metab. 2012;38 Suppl 3:S53–8.
48. Anderson CJ. The psychology of doing nothing: forms of decision avoidance result from reason and emotion. Psychol Bull. 2003;129:139–67.
49. Franc S, Daoudi A, Mounier S, Boucherie B, Laroye H, Peschard C, Dardari D, Juy O, Requeda E, Canipel L, Charpentier G. Telemedicine: what more is needed for its integration in everyday life? Diabet Med. 2011;37:S71–7.
50. Chabouis A, Berdugo M, Meas T, Erginay A, Laloi-Michelin M, Jouis V, Guillausseau PJ, M'bemba J, Chaine G, Slama G, Cohen R, Reach G, Marre M, Chanson P, Vicaut E, Massin P. Benefits of Ophdiat, a telemedical network to screen for diabetic retinopathy: a retrospective study in five reference hospital centres. Diabetes Metab. 2009;35:228–32.
51. Charpentier G, Benhamou PY, Dardari D, Clergeot A, Franc S, Schaepelynck-Belicar P, Catargi B, Melki V, Chaillous L, Farret A, Bosson JL, Penfornis A, TeleDiab Study Group. The Diabeo software enabling individualized insulin dose adjustments combined with telemedicine support improves HbA1c in poorly controlled type 1 diabetic patients: a 6-month, randomized, open-label, parallel-group, multicenter trial (TeleDiab 1 Study). Diabetes Care. 2011;34:533–9.
52. Reach G. The mental mechanisms of patient adherence to long term therapies, mind and care, Foreword by Pascal Engel, "Philosophy and Medicine" series, Springer, forthcoming.
53. Rosenthal MB, Frank RG, Zhonghe L, Epstein AM. Early experience with pay-for-performance: from concept to practice. JAMA. 2005;294:1788–93.
54. Lindenauer PK, Remus D, Roman S, Rothberg MB, Benjamin EM, Ma A, Bratzler DW. Public reporting and pay for performance in hospital quality improvement. N Engl J Med. 2007;356:486–96.
55. Lynagh MC, Sanson-Fisher RW, Bonevski B. What's good for the goose is good for the gander. Guiding principles for the use of financial incentives in health behavior change. Int J Behav Med. 2011. doi:10.1007/s12529-011-9202-5.
56. Glickman SW, Peterson ED. Innovative health reform models: pay-for-performance initiatives. Am J Manag Care. 2009;15:S300–5.
57. Elridge C, Palmer N. Performance-based payment: some reflections on the discourse, evidence and unanswered questions. Health Policy Plan. 2009;24:160–6.
58. Aron D, Pogach L. Specialists vs generalists in the era of pay for performance: "a plague o'both your houses !". Qual Saf Health Care. 2007;16:3–5.
59. Fink KS. Value-driven health care: proceed with caution. J Am Board Fam Med. 2008;21:458–60.
60. Baumann MH, Dellert E. Performance measures and pay for performance. Chest. 2006;129:188–91.
61. Van Herck P, De Smedt D, Annemans L, Remmen R, Rosenthal MB, Sermeus W. Systematic review: effects, design choices, and context of pay-for-performance in health care. BMC Health Serv Res. 2010;10:247.

62. De Bruin S, Baan CA, Struijs J. Pay-for performance in disease management: a systematic review of the literature. BMC Health Serv Res. 2011;11:272.
63. Scott A, Sivey P, Ait Ouakrim D, Willenberg L, Naccarella L, Furler J, Young D. The effect of financial incentives on the quality of health care provided by primary care physicians. Cochrane Database Syst Rev. 2011;(9):CD008451.
64. Houle SK, McAlister FA, Jackevicius CA, Chuck AW, Tsuyuki RT. Does performance-based remuneration for individual health care practitioners affect patient care?: a systematic review. Ann Intern Med. 2012;157:889–99.
65. Huang J, Yin S, Lin Y, Jiang Q, He Y, Du L. Impact of pay-for-performance on management of diabetes: a systematic review. J Evid Based Med. 2013;6(3):173–84. doi:10.1111/jebm.12052.
66. Le contrat d'amélioration des pratiques individuelles (CAPI). http://www.securite-sociale.fr/IMG/pdf/fiche_eclairage_maladie_capi_sept_2011.pdf. Accessed 7 Sept 2014.
67. Le contrat d'amélioration des pratiques individuelles (CAPI). http://www.securite-sociale.fr/IMG/pdf/fiche_eclairage_maladie_capi_sept_2011.pdf. Accessed 21 Apr 2014.
68. Sutton E, Wilson H, Kaboli PJ, Carter BL. Why physicians do not prescribe thiazide diuretics. J Clin Hypertens (Greenwich). 2010;12:502–7.
69. Agarwal R, Bills JE, Hecht TJ, Light RP. Role of home blood pressure monitoring in overcoming therapeutic inertia and improving hypertension control: a systematic review and meta-analysis. Hypertension. 2011;57:29–38.
70. Grant RW, Wald JS, Schnipper JL, Gandhi TK, Poon EG, Orav EJ, Williams DH, Volk LA, Middleton B. Practice-linked online personal health records for type 2 diabetes mellitus: a randomized controlled trial. Arch Intern Med. 2008;168:1776–82.
71. Portnoy DB, Scott-Sheldon LAJ, Johnson BT, Carey M. Computer-delivered interventions for health promotion and behavioral risk reduction: a meta-analysis of 75 randomized controlled trials, 1988–2007. Prev Med. 2008;47:3–16.
72. Thiboutot J, Stuckey H, Binette A, Kephart D, Curry W, Falkner B, Sciamanna C. A webbased patient activation intervention to improve hypertension care: study design and baseline characteristics in the web hypertension study. Contemp Clin Trials. 2010;3:634–46.
73. Groupes de pairs, le plaisir de se former ensemble. http://www.sfmg.org/groupe_de_pairs/. Accessed 9 Apr 2011.
74. Fiscella K, Volpe E, Winters P, Brown M, Idris A, Harren T. A novel approach to quality improvement in a safety-net practice: concurrent peer review visits. J Natl Med Assoc. 2010;102:1231–6.
75. van Bruggen R, Gorter K, Stolk R, Klungel O, Rutten G. Clinical inertia in general practice: widespread and related to the outcome of diabetes care. Fam Pract. 2009;26:428–36.
76. Kennedy AG, MacLean CD. Clinical inertia: errors of omission in drug therapy. Am J Health Syst Pharm. 2004;61:401–4.
77. Kirwin JL, Cunningham RJ, Sequist TD. Pharmacist recommendations to improve the quality of diabetes care: a randomized controlled trial. J Manag Care Pharm. 2010;16:104–13.
78. Carter BL, Bergus GR, Dawson JD, James PA, Bergus GR, Doucette WR, Chrischilles EA, Franciscus CL, Xu Y. A cluster randomized trial to evaluate physician/pharmacist collaboration to improve blood pressure control. J Clin Hypertens. 2008;10:260–71.
79. Elster J. Ulysses unbound, rationality, precommitments and constraints. Cambridge: Cambridge University Press; 2000.
80. Gollwitzer PM, Schaal B. Metacognition in action: the importance of implementation intentions. Pers Soc Psychol Rev. 1998;2:124–36.
81. Holton R. How is strength of will possible? In: Stroud S, Tappolet C, editors. Weakness of will and practical irrationality. Oxford: Clarendon; 2003. p. 39–67.
82. Searle J. Intentionality: an essay in the philosophy of mind. Cambridge, UK: Cambridge University Press; 1983.
83. Reach G. Role of habit in adherence to medical treatment. Diabet Med. 2005;22:415–20.
84. Proust J. La Nature de la volonté. Paris: Gallimard; 2005.

# References

85. Wise RA, Bozarth MA. A psychomotor stimkalnt theory of addiction. Psychol Rev. 1987;94:469–92.
86. Engel P. Préface à Paradoxes de l'irrationalité de Donald Davidson. Combas, L'Éclat; 1991.
87. Pears D. Motivated irrationality. South Bend: St Augustine's Press; 1998. p. 1.
88. Croskerry P. The cognitive imperative: thinking about how we think. Acad Emerg Med. 2000;7:1223–31.
89. Epstein RM, Siegel DJ, Silberman J. Self-monitoring in clinical practice: a challenge for medical educators. J Contin Educ Health Prof. 2008;28:5–13.
90. Bradley CP. Commentary: can we avoid bias? BMJ. 2005;330:784.
91. Phillips LS, Branch WT, Cook CB, Doyle JP, El-Kebbi IM, Gallina DL, Miller CD, Ziemer DC, Barnes CS. Clinical inertia. Ann Intern Med. 2001;135:825–34.
92. Wexler R, Elton T, Taylor CA, Pleister A, Feldman D. Physician reported perception in the treatment of high blood pressure does not correspond to practice. BMC Fam Pract. 2009;10:23.
93. Feinstein AR. The 'chagrin factor' and qualitative decision analysis. Arch Intern Med. 1985;145:1257–9.
94. Studdert DM, Mello MM, Sage WM, DesRoches CM, Peugh J, Zapert K, Brennan TA. Defensive medicine among high-risk specialist physicians in a volatile malpractice environment. JAMA. 2005;293:2609–17.
95. Frankfurt HG. The importance of what we care about. Cambridge, UK: Cambridge University Press; 1988.
96. Darwall S. Welfare and rational care. In: Princeton monographs in philosophy. Princeton: Princeton University Press; 2002.
97. Elster J. Alchemies of the mind: rationality of emotions. Cambridge: Cambridge University Press; 1999. p. 241.
98. Carver CS, Scheier MF, Segerstrom SC. Optimism. Clin Psychol Rev. 2010;30:879–89.
99. Higgins ET. Beyond pleasure and pain. Am Psychol. 1997;52:1280–300.
100. Veazie PJ, Qian F. A role for regulatory focus in explaining and combating clinical inertia. J Eval Clin Pract. 2011;17:1147–52.
101. Zikmund-Fisher BJ, Hofer TP, Klamerus ML, Kerr EA. First things first: difficulty with current medications is associated with patient willingness to add new ones. Patient 2009;2:221–231.
102. Nguyen GC, LaVeist TA, Harris ML, Datta LW, Bayless TM, Brant SR. Patient trust-in-physician and race are predictors of adherence to medical management in inflammatory bowel disease. Inflamm Bowel Dis. 2009;15:1233–9.
103. Thom DH, Campbell B. Patient-physician trust: an exploratory study. J Fam Pract. 1997;44: 169–76.
104. Thom DH. Stanford Trust Study Physicians, Physician behaviors that predict patient trust. J Fam Pract. 2001;50:323–8.
105. Zolnierek KB, Dimatteo MR. Physician communication and patient adherence to treatment: a meta-analysis. Med Care. 2009;47:826–34.
106. Origgi G. Qu'est-ce que la confiance Chemins philosophiques. Paris: Vrin; 2008. p. 7–8.
107. Hardin R. Trust and trustworthiness. New York: Russel Sage Foundation; 2004.
108. Spinoza. The Ethics, Part 4 of human bondage, Proposition LII, Proof and Corollary.
109. Spinoza. The Ethics, Part 3 on the origine and the nature of the emotions, Definitions XII and XIII.

# Conclusion: Time for Medical Reason

**8**

## Abstract

The phenomenon of clinical inertia of physicians who do not follow clinical practice guidelines was recognized recently and demands a reflection on the meaning of Evidence-Based Medicine. From an epistemological point of view, it is possible to consider Evidence-Based Medicine as a contemporary "invention" concomitant with those of patient education and the principle of autonomy in medicine. The fact that these three inventions were simultaneous allowed a balance between the first, establishing the state of knowledge of a medicine of diseases, and the latter two allowing the foundation of a person-centered medicine. But the three inventions are to a certain extent contradictory and their contradictions carry the seeds of patient nonadherence and physician clinical inertia, which are the revealing symptoms of these contradictions of modern medicine. This reflection allows one to understand the interest of "individualized" guidelines which will allow physicians to truly apply a sound practice of Evidence-Based Medicine: taking into account not only cohort-based science but also the individual character of any medical decision. Thus it is necessary to allow time for physician medical reason, which is to allow them to exercise their intellect: through this, medicine will keep its human dimension.

This investigation started from a surprising discovery: it occurs, in fact fairly often, that physicians do not apply clinical practice guidelines that are however widely disseminated. Of course, it is essential to distinguish true clinical inertia from situations where the physician's judgment recognizes that a guideline should not be applied to this patient she is faced with: this is not therefore clinical inertia but instead appropriate inaction. What's more, giving priority to the physician's clinical judgment is what the theory of Evidence-Based Medicine states time and again.

© Springer International Publishing Switzerland 2015
G. Reach, *Clinical Inertia: A Critique of Medical Reason*,
DOI 10.1007/978-3-319-09882-1_8

Thus, some authors even claimed that, in the case of diabetes treatment, physician clinical inertia is a "safeguard" for patients against questionable guidelines [1], questionable because there is little evidence that treatment intensification actually improves the cardiovascular prognosis of patients, and that on the contrary the ACCORD study [2] showed that excessive intensification increased the risk of mortality; but it would be an error to generalize this refusal to follow guidelines, which would actually come back to throwing the Evidence-Based Medicine baby out with the bathwater: this would be to forget that *most patients* benefit from intensive treatment of diabetes and that this must take place as of the diagnosis [3]; consequently, it is to *most patients'* advantage that their physicians follow guidelines, all while knowing that the HbA1c threshold where one must intervene should be discussed based on the context [4]: after all, this specific case could allow one to illustrate why medicine must stay an art.

Recently, a new form of guidelines have emerged in diabetes care: they must be *individualized*. This concept of "individualized guideline" may appear to be an oxymoron: wasn't the initial purpose of clinical practice guidelines to homogenize practices? How can a practitioner, faced with the uniqueness of the patient in front of her, find an answer to her questions in a text which is obliged to be generic? This question reveals the fact that medicine can be considered according to two scales, that of public health and that of day-to-day medicine, that of cohorts of patients and that of a person-centered medicine.

Clearly, the definition of a glycemic target in the treatment of diabetes must take into account the characteristics of patients, and this is what was missing in the ACCORD study, where an extreme intensification of treatment did not take into account the fact that the population concerned included patients that were elderly, diabetic for a long time, often polypathological, undoubtedly already having often a diseased heart. Taking into account the characteristics of the patient, is what one is now invited to do by the new, so-called individualized, guidelines published first in 2012 in an American-European consensus [5, 6], then in 2013 in France by the *Haute Autorité de Santé* [7]. The American-European consensus is particularly remarkable: the physician is invited to choose her target based on criteria which are not only biomedical, but biopsychosocial. In the end, if guidelines become more flexible because they are individualized, the issue of clinical inertia could almost disappear [8]. This clearly reveals the paradox of clinical inertia: it exists in relation to the nature of guidelines against which one contrasts the behavior of the physician.

But one should not see here a sleight of hand allowing one to eliminate what is in fact, lets recall, a reality and a major public health issue: indeed, it is one thing to not apply guidelines when this can be justified, what's more that's what the spirit of Evidence-Based Medicine recommends, it is another to not apply them *without reason*.

Nevertheless, one must come back to the Evidence: we have also observed that it occurs *very often* that physicians have good reasons to not apply guidelines. We have even cited a publication showing that in 93 % of cases these reasons could be validated by peers [9]. Moreover, one can recall the study by Crowley: physicians did not intensify antihypertensive treatment of a patient when they had received an alert informing them of elevated blood pressure readings; in the months that followed, they did not receive any more alerts regarding this patient, which appears to prove retrospectively that they were undoubtedly *right* [10].

Therefore, there seems to be discordance between the rationale on which Evidence-Based Medicine is based and what we have called "medical reason". This discordance can be described in two ways. On the one hand, if one follows Schön, who's book on the Reflective Practitioner we have cited [11], the methodology proposed by Evidence-Based Medicine falls under what he calls "Technical Rationality", meant to help the physician resolve clinical problems, even though the difficulty the physician is faced with is not situated in the resolution of problems, but in their formulation; yet for Schön, the formulation of problems does not fall under Technical Rationality, but instead under the Reflection-in-Action of the practitioner, that is to say an expertise which cannot be reduced to Technical Rationality: one can contrast, as Gabbay does, guidelines and mindlines, the guidelines which one asks the physician to follow and what her reason tells her [12]. On the other hand, guidelines represent general rules, while the therapeutic act is always applied to a singular patient, *in a certain context*.

## The Difference Between Two Dynamics

This led us to examine the differences between the two dynamics. At the end of this analysis, it appears to us indeed that Evidence-Based Medicine represents an attempt, falling within what Schön calls Technical Rationality, to allow a translation of data from clinical research into clinical practice guidelines. This "data" represents statistical results of studies which aim to provide a demonstration and, consequently, use the randomized clinical trial methodology which is definitely the best method that can do so *while avoiding biases*. This methodology has nevertheless the inconvenience of being based on construction of groups of "average patients" on which the comparisons will be based. Evidence-Based Medicine recognizes this and that is why it states time and again when it develops guidelines based on these studies that the physician, before applying them, should determine if the patient she is faced with resembles sufficiently the patients in the study. Indeed, the role of the physician, for its part, is no longer to give demonstrations but rather to treat individuals.

It's here that the notion of "individualized guideline" takes on its full value: the American-European consensus on diabetes treatment [5, 6] proposes a "less algorithmic" process than the previous guidelines. This is to recognize not only the uniqueness of all medical decisions, but also the fact that they cannot use an algorithmic process (an algorithm being a reasoning process in which a question has only one unique answer). The proposed process requires the physician to reflect on the uniqueness of the patient she is faced with, on her characteristics and her preferences (this is, what's more, what Evidence-Based Medicine had recommended from the start), in brief to use her medical reason, that is to say her intelligence [13].

But our analysis of mindlines, of medical reason seen from the perspective of the physician's mind, has also shown us that this is not a matter of a Kantian pure reason. On the one hand, it makes use of heuristics, which are *necessary* reasoning short-cuts given the limited nature of human rationality and the complexity of problems to be resolved, and which are therefore both useful and a possible source of cognitive biases. On the other hand, human reason is not purely cognitive: it also involves emotions (some refuse what's more to make the distinction between cognition and emotions, seeing in emotions a form of cognition) [14].

## Variability and Uncertainty

Thus, Evidence-Based Medicine has as its initial objective to remedy the *variability of medical practices* by disseminating clinical practice guidelines which, if they are applied, will make it that the greatest number of patients benefit from care considered as the best possible, based on the best scientific data available. The intention is to limit, in the minds of physicians, *the uncertainty* which leads to indecision, and therefore to clinical inertia.

Nevertheless, the production of Evidence which must lead to the development of these guidelines encounters *variability of another type*, *that of living phenomena*, perhaps itself relating to the variability of physical phenomena in general. This variability here constitutes an objective reality, existing in and of itself, independent of any observation, just as the sound of the wind in the trees exists even if nobody is in the forest to hear it. The calculation of conditional probabilities of Bayes' theorem (probability that the patient has the disease if the result of the test is positive) takes into account this variability. The same is true of statistical calculations which allow one, for example, to specify the number needed to treat to avoid a pathological event in randomized therapeutic trials. The role of investigators, in clinical trials which assess diagnostic tests and therapeutic options, is only to *describe*, if possible without bias, this variability and its consequences on the attributes of diagnostic tests and the effectiveness of treatment.

But uncertainty, which represents a major cause of decision avoidance described by Anderson in his review of the psychology of inaction (*The psychology of doing nothing*) [15], is not only caused by the intrinsic variability of all existing phenomena. One must add here another component that is due to the arrival of an *agent*, the physician, whom one asks to use generic Evidence, independent of all context, to answer the question asked by an issue, always new and unique, of true clinical practice. She must in fact engage in an *interpretation*, which introduces a new variability since it depends not only on a context but also on all that the physician thinks besides, on the trust that she can have regarding the source of information she is given, on her emotions, on the use of heuristics, etc. Perhaps one can thus see in the uncertainty which leads to the indecision of clinical inertia the result of the encounter between two kinds of variability, that, objective, of the Evidence observed, and that, subjective, of the physician which is confronted with this variability. It is precisely here, it seems to us, that is situated the encounter of two *dynamics*, that of Evidence-Based Medicine and that of the practitioner's medical reason, whose divergences can contribute to explain the gap between guidelines and clinical reality.

It is thus interesting to note, as Saarni and Gylling have done [16], that Evidence-Based Medicine can itself be seen as having two components: an *epistemic* component (the production of knowledge) and a *practical* component (the development of clinical practice guidelines). They note that there is often confusion between these two aspects when one speaks of Evidence-Based Medicine. They also show that the desire to limit the variability of medical practices, which is at the very origin of "the invention" of Evidence-Based Medicine in the history of contemporary medicine, has also a rationale which is not purely medical but also economic. This rationale could contribute, to a certain extent, to limit the autonomy of the physician and the patient in their capacities to choose: in the end, who decides, the physician, the patient, or the governing body who dictates the rules of best practice?

In summary, we can see the encounter between Evidence-Based Medicine and care as an encounter between "knowledge" produced *if possible* without bias, and a "practice" *necessarily* accompanied by bias, since it is no longer the practice that was conceived within the context of Evidence-Based Medicine that one is talking about, but rather the real practice, in the concrete sense of the term, that of the physician "in real life". In these conditions, the occurrence of the phenomenon which one calls clinical inertia is undoubtedly inevitable, since it's in light of the former that the latter will be described as appropriate or not.

## What to Do with Emotions?

One could reject this conclusion and say that physicians have learned or should learn to "manage their emotions". This is perhaps not so simple: one can recall the comment by Baumeister, suggesting that it is difficult for us to control our emotions, because our emotions are there to control us and contribute to the shaping of our cognition [17]. One can also cite an article regarding the management of the "hateful patient", published in 1978 in the *New England Journal Medicine*: "admitted or not, the fact remains that a few patients kindle aversion, fear, despair or even downright malice in their doctors. Emotional reactions to patients cannot simply be wished away, nor is it good medicine to pretend that they do not exist [18]."

It seems to us therefore more appropriate to suggest that what physicians must learn is *the existence* of their emotions and cognitive biases coming from the use of heuristics, because emotions and heuristics are an integral part of their medical reason, one would be tempted to say for better or for worse. This should be taught formally, undoubtedly very early in the medical studies curriculum. One should also teach future physicians to develop their capacity of psychological self-monitoring regarding their own behavior, such as it was described in detail by Epstein [19].

## An Epistemological Transition: What the Phenomena of Physician Clinical Inertia and Patient Nonadherence Reveal

One can propose that awareness, relatively late in coming, of the importance of patient nonadherence then of physician clinical inertia is the consequence of a true change of scenery that medicine experienced at the end of the last century. Indeed, at the end of the 1970–1990s, one first witnessed the emergence of Evidence-Based Medicine: medicine has become efficacious and has given itself the means to prove it, and it uses Evidence coming from its research to develop clinical practice guidelines. The very year, 1972, where Cochrane published his book [20], one sees the first publication on patient education which will allow the patient to benefit from this triumphant medicine: Leona Miller shows that one decreases through patient education the number of hospitalizations for acute complications from diabetes, the number of cases of ketoacidosis and the number of amputations [21]. But at the same time, in 1979, Tom Beauchamp and James Childress put forth the four principles of the new medical ethics: they propose to add to the two Hippocratic principles of beneficence and non-maleficence a principle of justice, and especially the principle of respect of patient autonomy [22].

This is clearly a complete change of scenery. Thus, just as Kant's clarification, in the eighteenth century, of the notion of autonomy represented a true "*invention*" of human thought, whose historical foundations Schneewind magnificently retraced [23], to recognize the existence in medical practice of a principle of autonomy also had an innovative nature which can literally be referred to as "inventive". Yet the same is true of the advent of Evidence-Based Medicine and patient education.

Of course, one can, in the coincidence of their "invention", see in Evidence-Based Medicine an answer from Medicine to "the invention" of the Principle of Autonomy in medicine, aiming to maintain its authority; in fact, Parker suggests on the contrary that Evidence-Based Medicine had the effect of replacing the historical and traditional authoritarianism of medicine by the better justified foundation of scientific and clinical revendications [24].

The same is true of the "invention" of patient education in medicine: beyond a transmission to the patient of information allowing her to acquire knowledge and skills, it was a matter of fundamentally recognizing as an obligation the right of patients to understand the significance of their disease and their treatment. The WHO has defined in 1998 four missions of patient education, taken up by the HPST law (loi *Hôpital, Patients, Santé, Territoires*) in the presentation of "specifications" to which all Patient Education Programs must answer [25]: (1) help patients to learn and teach patients to manage their treatment; (2) teach patients to manage the health, social and economic resources available; (3) help patients to manage their lifestyle; (4) take into account in patient education the educational, psychological and social dimensions of long-term management. We have shown elsewhere that each of these missions represents as many *innovations* in medicine [26]: this *educational posture* was in fact in theory not natural for the physician, if one considers that this consists for her of sharing her power with the patient, of accepting that medicine be carried out within a team of health care providers implementing multiple resources, of taking into account the lifestyle of the patient as a psychosocial being, finally of taking

# An Epistemological Transition: What the Phenomena of Physician Clinical Inertia

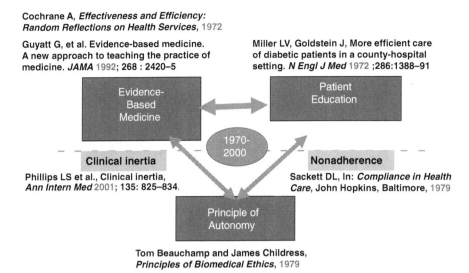

**Fig. 8.1** The epistemological transition of contemporary medicine: three "inventions"

into account the chronic nature of the disease that she treats. One notes the link which exists between "the invention" of the educational process in medicine and that of the Principle of Autonomy [27]; it is here that patient education aims to lead to what one calls patient empowerment [28].

These three "inventions", which were made concomitantly, are therefore linked and can be represented in the form of a triangulation (Fig. 8.1).

It was important that the three "inventions" took place at the same time, since this made a rebalancing possible: that of Evidence-Based Medicine, indeed, risked to found a *medicine of diseases*, essentially epidemiological. The inventions of patient education and the Principle of Autonomy allowed for the founding of an *individual medicine centered on the patient, as a person*.

Nevertheless, it is significant that it was also in the same year 1979 that the term compliance (nowadays referred to as adherence) entered into the medical vocabulary [29]: nonadherence intrigues since it represents an unexpected barrier to the efficiency of care. And in 2001, Phillips identified a second barrier: clinical inertia [30].

These barriers appear since the two sides of the triangle represented in Fig. 8.1 bring with them two contradictions, between, on the one side Evidence-Based Medicine and patient education, and on the other respect of autonomy. First, patient nonadherence can be seen as the consequence of the contradiction which exists, for the health care provider, between her desire for patient education and that of respecting the principle of patient autonomy: no treatment can be begun without the patient's consent; this means that the patient has the right to not be adherent, despite what patient education attempts to explain to her. Next, we can likewise see in clinical inertia the consequence of a conflict between Evidence-Based Medicine and respect of autonomy, that is to say, in a certain way, a medicine essentially centered on the person.

One understands thus why the two phenomena of patient nonadherence and clinical inertia are so linked, as this has emerged several times in this book. In one of the articles of the supplement of the journal *Médecine des Maladies Métaboliques* devoted to clinical inertia, Magalie Baudrant-Boga et al. ask if the true question is not in fact a question in common: "what level of risk-taking are patient and physician ready to take, when they deviate from clinical practice guidelines?" [31].

## Evidence-Based Medicine and Person-Centered Medicine

A *Person*? Of course, an autonomous person in the ethical sense of the term, that is to say having the skills to decide her destiny, having the capacity to evaluate her preferences and possibly to change them [32]; but also a person as an individual which perhaps has nothing to do with the "average patient" on which the study which served to develop the guidelines had been based: in particular, a person can be defined as a being having the capacity to evaluate her desires [33], that is to say to have preferences which can be defined as the value that the person gives to things [34]. Yet these values are absent *a priori* in the carrying out of clinical trials (except perhaps at the time of signing the informed consent documents). And here, consequently, is what the physician can implicitly say to herself: "Evidence-Based Medicine tells me to do this, but I do not do it, for such or such reason which my medical reason tells me *regarding this patient*, because the principle of autonomy tells me, for its part, that I must respect the fact that she is a person". This is what's more clearly what Evidence-Based Medicine recommends: one must not only ask if the patient one is faced with resembles the "average patient" of the study, but what's more, one must, in the end, inquire about her "values".

Medicine centered on the person as an individual, Aristotle said as much: "for the physician does not cure man, except in an incidental way, but Callias or Socrates or some other called by some such individual name, who happens to be a man. If, then, a man has the theory without the experience, and recognizes the universal but does not know the individual included in this, he will often fail to cure; for it is the individual that is to be cured" [35]. Person-centered medicine in its complete dimension is not only biomedical, but also and perhaps especially psychological and social: This is clearly the new, biopsychosocial, model of medicine whose advent George Engel had called for in 1977 [36].

## Educational Value of Guidelines

Again, one must insist upon the fact that one must be careful to not throw the Evidence-Based Medicine and clinical practice guidelines, one of the angles of the triangle, baby out with the bathwater, reintroducing an imbalance. Clinical practice guidelines represent in fact a need to clarify, at a given moment (since knowledge is not fixed) what was called in the past the state of the art, so that the greatest number of patients can benefit from it when appropriate, *which occurs nevertheless fairly often*, if not most often. This is why, one must teach medical students that they must go search out clinical practice guidelines, for example in France on the *Haute Autorité de Santé*'s website, since it is an effective means to give them access to controlled information, and for them to learn medicine; they must nevertheless read them critically, and it is important that they receive, early in their curriculum, training on how to exert their *medical reason*.

In summary, it well could be that clinical practice guidelines, which are *general rules*, can indeed have a major educational advantage (which what's more Evidence-Based Medicine demands: the very first publication using the word evidence-based medicine presented it as "a new way of *teaching* medicine" [37]), by representing *a necessary stage* in the development of the practitioner's "mindlines", and we have seen that they are what's more a component of these. One can recall here the five stages described in 1980 by Stuart E. Dreyfus and Hubert L. Dreyfus, which lead the novice to true mastery, for example while learning a language, the game of chess, or how to fly an airplane [38]: at first, the *novice* sees the game of chess as something independent of all context, using a few elementary notions, such as the respective values of the different pieces and the importance of positions on the chess board. Then, following the experience acquired by playing in actual situations, she becomes *competent*: she has learned to recognize recurrent situations, and this is the moment where one can teach her principles leading to an action faced with these situations. In their model, Dreyfus and Dreyfus call these principles "guidelines" and they indicate that they presuppose that the student can give them a meaning based on her experience. The following stage is that of *proficiency*: here, each situation is analyzed based on a goal, and the level reached allows one to give more or less importance to the elements observed; the problem is seen, not in a decomposed way, but globally, "holistically", in light of the reaching of a general goal. Then one arrives at *expertise*: up to then, the decision making process was still of an analytical type even if it had reached in the previous stage a holistic mode; now, each situation *intuitively* involves a decision. This has become possible because in the course of the previous stage, one had learned to associate the appropriate answer to situations. Finally, the authors propose that there is even a subsequent stage, that of *mastery*, in which decisions can be made in the absence of all conscious reasoning.

The disappearance of the explicit intervention of rules in the reasoning process is described in another text by Hubert Dreyfus: "if one asks an expert how she has reasoned, which rules she has used, she will not be able to answer, because, simply, the expert does not use rules! If one asks for rules from an expert, one forces her in fact to regress to the level of a beginner and to put forth the rules which she still remembers, but which she no longer uses" [39]. It suffices to think of the way in which we start our car in the morning, without having to "decompose" the different gests that we have learned at driving school, then drive all the way to our workplace stopping at every red light, even though we are completely absorbed in our thoughts. This is not the mechanism of habit which we have mentioned in the previous chapter. It seems rather that the rules that we have learned have finished by, to adopt the expression by John Searle, "receding into the Background" [40], this set of presuppositions which allows our mental system to function. Or, if one likes, this relates to the fact that, according to Daniel Kahneman, the human mind more often uses the fast, intuitive, system of thought (System 1) over the slow, analytical, system of thought (System 2) [41].

Evocation of the Dreyfus and Dreyfus learning model suggests that there could therefore exist a stage, expertise, were one no longer use "rules". Nevertheless, these were *necessary, at a given moment, in the learning process*; afterwards decisions can be made without using them, at least explicitly. If one comes back to the issue of a professional practice, this is also what Schön noted when he stated that, in action, the "practitioner" uses tacit knowledge which she can at times not express [11].

The preceding does not mean, of course, that, in her practice, the physician *never again* uses the rules when she makes a decision: in fact, as we have said, guidelines are an integral part of her mindlines. The rules still exist in her mind, as something tacit. But, through the reflectivity of which Schön speaks, the "reflective practitioner" has integrated them in her practice, through the reflection which she has conducted before, during, and after the course of her action. Therefore they no longer exist as such but within a contextual framework, and the physician now knows when and how she must use them (as, what's more, Evidence-Based Medicine has continued to state time and again). In an article published in the same supplement of the journal *Médecine des Maladies Métaboliques*, Claude Attali et al. proposed that development of the physician's reflective posture can represent a path to overcome clinical inertia [42]. It appears to us that this is exactly what Epstein et al. have called "self-monitoring" [19].

## Tacit Nature of Knowledge and Holistic Base of "Mindlines"

Likewise, and on a much broader level, there are things which we know without knowing that we know them. This applies to "propositional" (or, as Searle states, "Intentional" [40]) knowledge, this knowledge which has a content (I know that): as the philosopher Pascal Engel proposes in his book *Va Savoir, de la connaissance en général*, when I say, for example, that I know that I have a hand, I need neither to know that I know it, nor to be able to say how I know it [43].

Moreover, Engel shows that knowledge is not necessarily completely *exact*; in fact, one "knows" something with "certitude" if one tells oneself that one could not have easily made a mistake: "knowledge contains a variable margin of approximation or error. Approximate knowledge, to adopt the term by Bachelard, is possible: in science or in common sense, knowledge accepts a certain margin of error, based on a margin of probability, without coming back to a Cartesian conception of certitude, in which one could never be refuted" [44]. One can also quote him in the evocation he makes on the relationship between knowledge and action: "another consideration in favor of the principle of certitude and which agrees well with that of the margin of error is the close link between knowledge and action [...] Just as my beliefs can be sure without however excluding a margin of error, my actions can be successful without however excluding a margin of error. If I intend to grab a glass, my gesture is such that there could be diverse similar movements in close possible words, which would lead to the same result. It suffices that my action is successful" [43].

In the same line of thinking and also very generally, the philosopher Frank Ramsey (1903–1930) put forth two theorems on belief: the more the content of my belief is true, the more the actions that I could be led to perform based on this belief will be successful (the more it is true that yellow mushrooms are edible, the less I take a risk by eating them); and the more I believe something with conviction, the more I will be inclined to act based on this belief (the more I am convinced that yellow mushrooms are edible, the more I will be inclined to eat them) [45, 46].

These *philosophical* notions, which integrate the variability in the theories of the rationality of action, obviously apply directly to the question treated here: the more it is *true* that intensifying the treatment is good for the patient's health (what such and such large randomized clinical study has shown, with a certain possible degree of error), the more that applying this guideline has a chance of being beneficial. But, what's more, according to Ramsey's second theorem, the more the physician is convinced that it is beneficial to prescribe the medication, the more she will be inclined to apply the guideline which tells her to do so. One understands that it is good that the study on which the guideline is based was published in a major journal, or else that the physician's attention was drawn to this study or to the guideline by an *opinion leader* whom she trusts.

It is therefore based on *all that she "knows" with more or less conviction*, on what was described under the term "mindlines", that the physician makes her decisions: this is a process which is not analytical but profoundly holistic; what's more, in the learning model by Dreyfus and Dreyfus which we have evoked, the holistic nature of decisions is noted starting from the stage of "proficiency" [38]. It's through this holistic approach that the physician can deal with the five challenges, described by Schön, which she encounters in her current practice: the challenges of complexity, uncertainty, instability, uniqueness of each decision, and value conflict [11].

## Appropriate Inaction and "True" Clinical Inertia: In Both Cases, Actions

One should come back to the notion of *appropriate inaction*. It occurs often, in fact, that the true medical error is not the error *of omission* – I did not apply the guideline of "best" practice – but rather an error *of commission*: I applied it, yet the error was precisely to think that it applied to this patient I had in front of me. Thus, just as it is essential to teach future physicians to read a medical article critically, one must teach them to develop the same critical thinking regarding the concept of "guidelines": (1) they have but a general nature; (2) they are often based on studies that have shown improvement in an *intermediate* clinical (blood pressure) or biological (HbA1c, cholesterol) parameter, while what is important, are the "morbimortality" criteria (number of events, death rate); (3) the medical paradigms on which they are based can change: let's take for example the idea of "lower is better" which is challenged by the J-curves that can be observed for many parameters such as glycemia or blood pressure; or else the consequences of the appearance of new therapeutic classes; even the fact that one can some day change therapeutic paradigm, for example in diabetes treatment by proposing an earlier introduction of insulin [47]; (4) especially, as we have continuously stated, they are only valid for patients which truly resemble the "average patient" that was included in the large studies on which they were founded, particular caution needing to be used for elderly patients, with multiple diseases and often "polymedicated". As Tonelli [48], whom we have extensively cited, states, clinicians *must be trained and allowed to deviate from clinical practice guidelines and protocols*; they must know to use physiopathological reasoning; in a word, they must know to safeguard the supremacy of their clinical sense.

We have seen throughout this book that one must therefore clearly distinguish "appropriate inaction" and "true clinical inertia": there is clearly on the one side the fact of not following a clinical practice guideline in such a way that this can be justified or because the "reflective practitioner" feels, intuitively, without necessarily being able to explain why, that another decision is appropriate – in this sense, Halimi and Attali were right to say that this "appropriate inaction" is indeed an action [49]; but on the other side, there is "true clinical inertia", that which is based on nothing, even if it also has mental mechanisms, which we have tried to describe, which make it that preference is given to the *status quo*.

Yet *doing nothing* within the context of this true clinical inertia *also represents an action*, whose mechanism was represented in Fig. 6.1 of Chap. 6 (page 74). But here, beliefs are biased, emotions are the cause, as Christine Tappolet states [50], of weakness of will, or, as Vasco Correia proposed, of denial, what philosophers call self-deception [51]: denial of the gravity of the patient's situation or denial, for the physician, of her own clinical inertia. Finally, the role of resources intervenes in a major way, since we have insisted upon the effect of lack of time as a determinant of true clinical inertia – the physician did not have the time to exert her medical reason.

## Overcoming True Clinical Inertia

As we have demonstrated, the notion of clinical inertia is born of the observation of the existence of a "gap" between guidelines and their practical use, a gap whose breadth we have described in the first part of this book, and one must not deny that it occurs at least sometimes, if not often, that these divergences cannot be justified. This *true clinical inertia* is always open to criticism [52] in the sense that it can have deleterious consequences on the health or even the life of patients, without speaking of consequences in terms of health care expenditure, and one must therefore try to correct it, or rather try to prevent its occurrence.

One understands therefore the justification of the desire to improve the situation through organizational measures, and they can be effective: for example, in the case of the management of diabetes in France, the ENTRED study highlighted a clear improvement – even if a lot of work still needs to be done, between 2001 and 2007, not only in follow-up procedures, but also in treatment intensification of diabetes, hypertension and hypercholesterolemia [53, 54]. It is therefore likely that things are improving. We have also cited a study showing that physicians having completed their MD after 1995 were more often compliant with clinical practice guidelines [55], and one can think that there will be a positive effect of the new medical culture which is establishing itself and the necessary reorganization of the health care system which it involves.

Among these organizational measures, one understands the purpose of current experiments with physician incentives through "Pay for Performance" type systems. It is a matter of increasing the efficiency of care by fundamentally improving access to care, since *true clinical inertia* represents a barrier to this access. Yet Woolf and Johnson have clearly shown that increasing access to care would be more effective than the development of a new medication: imagine a disease which causes 100,000 deaths per year, with a medication A that saves 20 % of patients, therefore 20,000 people. But if medication A is prescribed to only 80 % of patients which could benefit from it, it will save only 16,000 people. One would need a medication B saving 25 % of lives to have the same effect (to save 20,000 people) when it is given to 80 % of patients, as medication A if it were prescribed to everyone. Now, if medication A is prescribed to only 60 % of patients, medication B should save 33.3 % of patients: the greater the gap of lack of prescription, the more the increase in the effectiveness of medications to compensate for it becomes important, at levels which may be unrealistic: it should thus be more profitable to tackle the problem of access to care than to develop new medications [56].

## Time for Medical Reason

Improving access to care by overcoming clinical inertia, there is no denying that this takes time, and first of all organizational time: one has cited a study showing that among the Centers of the Veteran Health Administration, it was those which had devoted resources to the implementation of guidelines which were the most efficient [57]; but especially, individual time on the part of the physician. We have seen as a *leitmotif* the impact of appointments that are too short, especially when faced with "competing demands" [58], and we have even been able to outline the mental mechanisms of the effect of time on "medical reason". Medical shortages which currently prevail must imperatively be resolved if one actually wishes to tackle the problem of clinical inertia, and one must invent new organizational means – for example through the use of telemedicine – to give physicians time. Otherwise, their time being limited, one can fear that that which physicians consecrate to trying to obtain good indicators within the context of Pay for Performance might be taken to the detriment of other medical tasks.

In the volume *Thinking* of *The Life of the Mind*, Hannah Arendt described *the moment when we think* as the present instant where, "in the gap between past and future, we find our place in time" [59]. If the physician cannot give time in the present to find the time to think that her appointment is in fact "this gap between the past and the future" of the history of her patient's disease as she understands it, she will stop thinking of the future, will hide in the past, and this would be clinical inertia.

It is therefore indispensable that reorganization of the health care system involves an in-depth reflection on medical time. Medical time is not only that of the appointment. It is perhaps especially the *time for reflection* (which can take place after the appointment). This reflection on medical time will become particularly important if one generalizes the principle of individualized guidelines, as this is starting to be done in diabetes care. Yet all the preceding suggests that this principle, far from being an oxymoron, represents the foundation of what evidence-based medicine should have never ceased to be: an intelligent medicine.

Indeed one hopes that physicians, having been incited to follow clinical practice guidelines, never find here cookbooks which would allow them to inexpensively (and even with the benefits of Pay for Performance) do without their *medical reason*: to avoid the biases of these short-cuts which are heuristics, one would use other *reasoning short-cuts* clearly presenting more dangers if they were used as such.

One must recognize the importance of taking into account the context in all decisions: only human reason is able to make it that guidelines coming from the "new way to practice medicine" are applied only when they should be. In the field of care as in other fields, human reason is made of knowledge, skills, experience and an indescribable capacity of reflectivity which allows it to self-construct based on not only experience, but also heuristics and emotions which, even if they are at times a source of bias, are *necessary* components of this permanent self-construction. This is what we have called *medical reason*, whose complexity we have attempted to describe. It's through it that medicine will be able to, by remaining a person-centered medicine, keep its human dimension.

## References

1. Giugliano D, Esposito K. Clinical inertia as a clinical safeguard. JAMA. 2011;305:1591–2.
2. Gerstein HC, Miller ME, Byington RP, Goff Jr DC, Bigger JT, Buse JB, Cushman WC, Genuth S, Ismail-Beigi F, Grimm Jr RH, Probstfield JL, Simons-Morton DG, Friedewald WT. Action to Control Cardiovascular Risk in Diabetes Study Group. Effects of intensive glucose lowering in type 2 diabetes. N Engl J Med. 2008;358:2545–59.
3. Mohan AV, Phillips LS. Clinical inertia and uncertainty in medicine. JAMA. 2011;306:383.
4. Ismail-Beigi F, Moghissi E, Tiktin M, Hirsch IB, Inzucchi SE, Genuth S. Individualizing glycemic targets in type 2 diabetes mellitus: implications of recent clinical trials. Ann Intern Med. 2011;154:554–9.
5. Inzuchi SE, Bergenstal RM, Buse JB, et al. Management of hyperglycemia in type2 diabetes: a patient-centered approach. Position Statement of the American Diabetes Association (ADA) and the European Association for the Study of Diabetes (EASD). Diabetologia. 2012;55:1577–96.
6. Inzuchi SE, Bergenstal RM, Buse JB, et al. Management of hyperglycemia in type2 diabetes: a patient-centered approach. Position Statement of the American Diabetes Association (ADA) and the European Association for the Study of Diabetes (EASD). Diabetes Care. 2012;35:1364–79.
7. Stratégie médicamenteuse du contrôle glycémique du diabète de type 2. http://www.has-sante.fr/portail/jcms/c_1022476/fr/strategie-medicamenteuse-du-controle-glycemique-du-diabete-de-type-2. Accessed 21 Apr 2014.
8. Esposito K, Ceriello A, Giugliano D. Does personalized diabetology overcome clinical uncertainty and therapeutic inertia in type 2 diabetes? Endocrine. 2013;44:343–5.
9. Persell SD, Dolan NC, Friesema EM, Thompson JA, Kaiser D, Baker DW. Frequency of inappropriate medical exceptions to quality measures. Ann Intern Med. 2010;152:225–31.

# References

10. Crowley MJ, Smith VA, Olsen MK, Danus S, Oddone EZ, Bosworth HB, Powers BJ. Treatment intensification in a hypertension telemanagement trial. Clinical inertia or good clinical judgment? Hypertension. 2011;58:552–8.
11. Schön DA. The reflective practioner. How professionals think in action. New York: Basic Books; 1983.
12. Gabbay J, le May A. Evidence based guidelines or collectively constructed "mindlines"? Ethnographic study of knowledge management in primary care. BMJ. 2004;329:1013–7.
13. Reach G. Clinical inertia, uncertainty and individualized guidelines. Diabetes Metab. 2014. pii:S1262-3636(14)00003-2. doi:10.1016/j.diabet.2013.12.009.
14. Oum R, Lieberman D. Emotion is cognition: an information-processing view of the mind. In: Vohs KD, Baumeister RF, Loewenstein G, editors. Do emotions help or hurt decision making. New York: Russell Sage Foundation; 2007. p. 117–32.
15. Anderson CJ. The psychology of doing nothing: forms of decision avoidance result from reason and emotion. Psychol Bull. 2003;129:139–67.
16. Saarni SI, Gylling HA. Evidence based medicine guidelines: a solution to rationing or politics disguised in science? J Med Ethics. 2004;30:171–5.
17. Baumeister RF, Vohs KD, DeWall CN, Zhang L. How emotion shapes behavior: feedback, anticipation, and reflexion, rather than direct causation. PSPR. 2007;11:167–203.
18. Groves JE. Taking care of the hateful patient. N Engl J Med. 1978;298:883–7.
19. Epstein RM, Siegel DJ, Silberman J. Self-monitoring in clinical practice: a challenge for medical educators. J Cont Educ Health Prof. 2008;28:5–13.
20. Cochrane AL. Effectiveness and efficiency: random reflections on health services. London: Nuffield Provincial Hospitals Trust; 1972. (réédition 1989, Royal Society of Medicine Press, London).
21. Miller LV, Goldstein J. More efficient care of diabetic patients in a county-hospital setting. N Engl J Med. 1972;286:1388–91.
22. Beauchamp TF, Childress JL. Principles of biomedical ethics. New York: Oxford; 1979.
23. Schneewind JB. The invention of autonomy. Cambridge/New York: Cambridge University Press; 1998.
24. Parker M. False dichotomies: EBM, clinical freedom, and the art of medicine. J Med Ethics Med Humanit. 2005;31:23–30.
25. Arrêté du 2 août 2010 relatif aux compétences requises pour dispenser l'éducation thérapeutique du patient. Journal Officiel de la République Française n° 0178, 4 août 2010, texte 30.
26. Reach G. Une Éducation Thérapeutique sans posture n'est qu'une imposture. In: Éducation Thérapeutique, La Mise en Oeuvre, Synthèse Pratique Mise au point 2011–2012, Grimadi A, ed., Éditions Scientifiques LC; 2011. p. 11–3.
27. Reach G. Patient autonomy in chronic care: solving a paradox. Patient Prefer Adherence. 2013;8:15–24.
28. Funnell MM, Anderson RM, Arnold MS, Barr PA, Donnelly M, Johnson PD, Taylor-Moon D, White NH. Empowerment: an idea whose time has come in diabetes education. Diabetes Educ. 1991;17:37–41.
29. Sackett DL. Compliance in health care. Baltimore: John Hopkins; 1979.
30. Phillips LS, Branch WT, Cook CB, Doyle JP, El-Kebbi IM, Gallina DL, Miller CD, Ziemer DC, Barnes CS. Clinical inertia. Ann Intern Med. 2001;135:825–34.
31. Baudrant-Boga M, Allenet B. Inertie clinique: et le patient dans tout ça? Médecine des Maladies Métaboliques. 2011;5 Suppl 2:S76–80.
32. Dworkin G. The theory and practice of autonomy. Cambridge/New York: Cambridge University Press; 1988.
33. Frankfurt H. Freedom of the will and the concept of a person. J Philos. 1971;68:5–20.
34. Lewis D. Dispositional theories of values. Proc Aristotelian Soc. 1989;63:113–37.
35. Aristote. Métaphysique, traduction de Marie-Paule Duminil et Annick Jaulin, "GF Flammarion", Flammarion, Paris; 2008, A, 1, 981a [15, 20]. p. 72–3.
36. Engel GL. The need for a new medical model: a challenge for biomedicine. Science. 1977;196:129–36.

37. Guyatt G, et al. Evidence-based medicine. A new approach to teaching the practice of medicine. JAMA. 1992;268:2420–5.
38. Dreyfus SE, Dreyfus HL. A five-stage model of the mental activities involved in directed skill acquisition (1980), reprinted. Bull Sci Technol Soc. 2004;24:177–81.
39. Dreyfus HL. La portée philosophique du connexionnisme. In: Introductions aux sciences cognitives, sous la direction de D. Andler, 1992. p. 352–73.
40. Searle J. Intentionality, an essay in the philosophy of mind. Cambridge/New York: Cambridge University Press; 1983.
41. Kahneman D. Thinking, fast and slow. London: Allen Lane; 2011.
42. Attali C, Le Breton J, Bercier S, Chartier S. "Arrêtez de tirer sur le pianiste !" Le point de vue du médecin généraliste sur l'inertie thérapeutique. Médecine des Maladies Métaboliques. 2011;5 Suppl 2:S69–75.
43. Engel P. Va Savoir, de la Connaissance en général, Hermann, 2007.
44. Engel P. Vérité, croyance et connaissance: propos d'un béotien dogmatique. In: Wald Lasowski A. Pensées pour le XXIème siècle, Fayard, 2008.
45. Ramsey F. Logique, Philosophie et Probabilités, Traduction sous la direction de Pascal Engel et Mathieu Marion, "Mathesis". Paris: Vrin; 2003. p. 164.
46. Dokic C, Engel P. Ramsey, Vérité et succès, "Philosophies". Paris: Presses Universitaires de France; 2001. p. 71.
47. Hsu WC. Consequences of delaying progression to optimal therapy in patients with type 2 diabetes not achieving glycemic goals. South Med J. 2009;102:67–76.
48. Tonelli MR. Integrating clinical research into clinical decision making. Ann Ist Super Sanita. 2011;47:26–30.
49. Halimi S, Attali C. L'inertie thérapeutique dans le diabète de type 2: la comprendre sans la banaliser. Médecine des Maladies Métaboliques. 2011;5 Suppl 2:S62–8.
50. Tappolet C. Emotions and the intelligibility of akratic actions. In: Stroud S, Tappolet C, editors. Weakness of will and practical irrationality. Oxford: Clarendon; 2003.
51. Correia V. La Duperie de soi et le problème de l'irrationalité: Des Illusions de l'esprit à la faiblesse de la volonté. Éditions Universitaires Européennes, 2010.
52. Reach G. La véritable inertie clinique: une attitude toujours critiquable. Médecine des Maladies Métaboliques. 2011;5 Suppl 2:S57–61.
53. Fagot-Campana A, Fosse S, Roudier C, Romon I, Penfornis A, Lecomte P, Bourdel-Marchasson I, Chantry M, Deligne J, Fournier C, Poutignat N, Weill A, Paulier A, Eschwège E, pour le Comité Scientifique Entred. Caractéristiques, risque vasculaire et complications des personnes diabétiques en France métropolitaine: d'importantes évolutions entre Entered 2001 et Entred 2007. Bull Epidemiol Hebd. 2009;42–43:436–40.
54. Robert J, Roudier C, Poutignat N, Fagot-Campana A, Weill A, Rudnichi A, Thammavong N, Fontbonne A, Detournay B, pour le Comité Scientifique Entred. Prise en charge des personnes diabétiques de type 2 en France en 2007 et tendances par rapport à 2001. Bull Epidemiol Hebd. 2009;42–43:455–60.
55. Sammer CE, Lykens K, Singh KP. Physician characteristics and the reported effect of evidence-based practice guidelines. Health Serv Res. 2008;43:569–81.
56. Woolf SH, Johnson RE. The break-even point: when medical advances are less important than improving the fidelity with which they are delivered. Ann Fam Med. 2005;3:545–52.
57. Ward MM, Yankey JW, Vaughn TE, BootsMiller BJ, Flach SD, Welke KF, Pendergast JF, Perlin J, Doebbeling BN. Physician process and patient outcome measures for diabetes care: relationships to organizational characteristics. Med Care. 2004;42:840–50.
58. Parchman ML, Pugh JA, Romero RL, Bowers KW. Competing demands or clinical inertia: the case of elevated glycosylated hemoglobin. Ann Fam Med. 2007;5:196–201.
59. Arendt H. The Life of the Mind, vol 1: Thinking. New York: Harvest Books; 1978. p. 209–10.

# By the Same Author

The Mental Mechanisms of Patient Adherence to Long Term Therapies, Mind and Care, Foreword by Pascal Engel, Philosophy and Medicine, Springer, 2015.

© Springer International Publishing Switzerland 2015
G. Reach, *Clinical Inertia: A Critique of Medical Reason*,
DOI 10.1007/978-3-319-09882-1

# Index

**A**

Adherence, x, xii, xv, xvi, 2, 3, 5, 17, 22, 24, 36–40, 61, 68, 73, 74, 89, 91, 93, 100–102, 110, 112–114, 127
Algorithmic, 123
Anderson, C.J., 104, 124
Anderson, G.M., 91, 92
Anticipated emotions, 85, 86, 90
Arendt, H., 133
Aristotle, 128
Asthma, 23, 34, 37, 38, 63
Attali, C., 68, 130, 132
Autonomy, 126, 127
Availability heuristic, 77
Awareness–Agreement–Adoption–Adherence model, 38–39

**B**

Bachelard, G., 130
Bachimont, J., 59
Barriers, 5, 20, 23, 24, 34, 37–40, 60, 81, 101, 127
Baumeister, R.F., ix, 86, 87, 125
Bayes, T., 52, 53, 66, 68, 77, 78, 80, 81, 111, 124
Bayes' theorem, 51–54
Beauchamp, T.F., 126
Beddoe, T., 45
Berlowitz, D.R., 15, 16, 20
Bias, xii, 60, 76–84, 91, 93, 99, 108, 110, 111, 124, 125, 134
Biopsychosocial, 122, 128

**C**

Cabana, M.D., 5, 34, 36–38, 101
Campbell, N.C., 62
Cardiovascular, 21

Cardiovascular risk factors, xv
Carver, C.S., 113
Centered on the patient, 127
Chagrin, 84, 88, 111
Childress, 126
Choudhry, N.K., 88
Chronic disease, 98, 104
Claude Bernard, 58
Clinical inertia, ix, xv, 2, 3, 5–10, 14–21, 23–25, 31–36, 38–42, 60, 61, 65, 67, 68, 75, 78, 80–82, 84, 88–93, 97, 99, 101–114, 121, 122, 124–128, 130–133
Clinical practice guidelines, 1, 3, 5–8, 22, 31, 34, 36, 46, 48–50, 55, 59, 92, 99, 101, 105, 111, 121–126, 128, 132–134
Cochrane, A.L., 7, 46, 49, 100, 106, 126
Communication, 35, 49, 113
Competing demands, 18–20, 32, 39, 41, 104, 108, 109, 133
Complete arrhythmia, atrial fibrillation, 23
Compliance, xi, xvi, 2, 7, 9, 20, 22, 36, 38–40, 60, 68, 75, 80, 81, 100, 101, 127
Concern, 112
Contrats d'Amélioration des Pratiques Individuelles (CAPI), 107
Coordinated Health Care Plan, 104
Correia, V., 132
Croskerry, P., 77, 81, 83, 110
Crowley, M.J., 122

**D**

Damasio A.R., 83, 85
Darwall, S., 112
Defensive medicine, 111
Depression, 24, 35, 39
Descartes, R., 83
Desire, 40, 67, 74, 90, 97, 105, 109, 112, 113, 125, 127, 132

© Springer International Publishing Switzerland 2015
G. Reach, *Clinical Inertia: A Critique of Medical Reason*,
DOI 10.1007/978-3-319-09882-1

# Index

Diabetes, xii, xv, 1, 5, 6, 8, 9, 13–22, 32–35, 41, 59, 62, 67, 81, 99, 100, 102, 103, 105–108, 112, 122, 123, 126, 132, 134
Disadvantaged, 17, 34, 74
Disease Management, 104, 106
Dreyfus, S.E., 129–131
Dreyfus, H.L., 129–131

### E

Education, 21, 33, 97–102, 126
Einstein, A., 58–59, 84, 114
Elster, J., 108, 112
Emotional reversal, 98, 111–114
Emotions, x, 73–75, 78–93, 97–99, 110–114, 124, 125, 132, 134
Engel, G.L., 128
Engel, P., ix, 130
Epstein, A.M., 110
Epstein, R.M., 125, 130
Evidence-based medicine, ix, xi, 1, 3, 7, 25, 37, 42, 45–68, 80–83, 88, 92, 93, 97, 99, 121–130, 134
Evidence practice gap, 7–8

### F

Facilitator, 98
Fear, 19, 32, 36, 38, 63, 85, 86, 88, 91, 99, 102, 103, 111, 112, 114, 125, 133
Feelings, 84–86, 112
Feinstein, A.R., 56, 60, 61, 63, 88, 111
Framing, 79, 82
Frankfurt, H., 112

### G

Gabbay, J., 67, 123
Generalizability, 62
Gollwitzer, P.M., 109
Goodhart's law, 106
Guidelines, xii, 1–3, 5–10, 13–25, 31, 32, 34, 36–38, 40, 42, 46–47, 49, 50, 56, 59, 60, 62, 63, 66, 67, 80, 81, 90, 92, 97–101, 103, 104, 111, 122–125, 128–134
Guyatt, G., 7, 46, 56

### H

Habit, 38, 109–110, 129
Halimi, S., 68, 132
Hateful patient, 125
Haute Autorité de Santé, ix, 1, 7, 47, 122, 129
Haynes, R.B., 49

HbA1c, xv, 2, 6, 8, 14, 16–19, 34, 41, 100, 102–104, 108, 122, 131
Health care expenditure, 3, 36, 106, 132
Health care providers, xv, xvi, 5–6, 17, 101, 102, 126
Heart failure, 21–22
Heisenberg, W., 58
Heuristics, 76, 78, 80–84, 88, 89, 110
Higgins, E.T., 40, 89, 113
Hôpital, Patients, Santé, Territoires (HPST), 105, 126
Horwitz, R.L., 56, 60, 61, 63
Howick, J., 56
HPST. *See* Hôpital, Patients, Santé, Territoires (HPST)
Hypercholesterolemia, 1, 2, 9, 14, 17, 18, 21, 32, 39, 41, 99, 108, 133
Hyperlipidemia, 21
Hypertension, xv, xvi, 1, 2, 6, 13, 15, 17, 18, 20–22, 32, 33, 35, 41, 62, 63, 101, 103, 106–108, 111, 133

### I

Implementation intention, 109
Inaction, xii, 10, 14, 24–25, 63, 68, 88, 92, 93, 106, 121, 124, 131–132
Incentive, 105–108
Inclusion criteria, 61–62
Indecision, 102, 124
Individualized guidelines, 68, 122, 123, 134
Intentional, 74, 109
Intention to treat, 61
Internet, 37, 49, 107
Inventions, 127

### K

Kahneman, D., ix, xi, 76, 78, 79, 88, 130
Kamhi, A.G., 50, 62
Kerr, E.A., 15, 33
Knowledge, xv, 7, 36–39, 45, 49, 52, 60, 62, 64–66, 73–75, 97, 99, 125, 126, 128, 130–131, 134
Knowledge–Attitude–Behavior–Result model, 36–37
Kuhn, T.S., 56
Kulkarni, A., 57

### L

Lack of time, 32
Laplace, P.S. de, 52

# Index

LDL-cholesterol, 2, 10, 15, 16, 18, 21, 100, 102–104
le May, A., 67
Loewenstein, G., x, 84–86

## M

McAlister, F.A., 60
Mechanisms, xvi, 3, 25, 73, 75, 80, 83, 87, 91, 92, 99, 132, 133
Medical error, 8–9
Medical reason, 3, 68, 73–93, 99, 110, 114, 121–134
Meta-analysis, xv, 100, 106, 107, 114
Mickan, S., 40
Miles, R.W., 81
Mindlines, 66–68, 75, 123, 124, 129–131

## N

Nonadherence, x, 2, 3, 6, 7, 10, 17, 20, 24, 31, 32, 35–37, 40, 41, 75, 82, 89–93, 99, 102, 105, 110, 111, 114, 126–128
Noncompliance, 6, 31, 38, 75
Nurses, 103, 105, 108, 111

## O

O'Connor, P.J., 6, 35, 100
Okonofua, E.C., 6, 14, 15
Omission, 9, 23, 40, 41, 88, 89, 91, 131
Opinion leader, 131
Opinion leaders, 67, 100
Osler, W., 7
Osteoporosis, 24–25

## P

Pain, 39–41, 73, 74, 77, 88, 89, 112, 114
Paradigm, 25, 33, 56–58, 62–63, 132
Parchman, M.L., 32
Parker, M., 60, 66, 126
Pasteur, L., 58
Pathman, D.E., 38, 39
Pay for Performance, 105–107, 133, 134
Peers, x, 10, 38, 108, 122
Person, 128
Pharmacists, 108
Phillips, L., 2, 5, 9, 10, 21, 32, 33, 35, 68, 84, 100, 103, 111, 127
Philosopher, ix, 82, 109, 110, 112, 114, 130, 131
Philosophy of mind, 108–109

Physician Guideline Compliance Model, 39–40
PICO, 48, 65
Polypharmacy, 10, 67
Positivism, 64
Preferences, x, 38, 46, 47, 49, 54, 60, 62, 65, 66, 68, 76, 92, 123, 128
Probability, xvi, 7, 14, 50–55, 57, 76–78, 85, 88, 124, 130
Promotion and prevention focuses, 41
Proof, xv, 6, 7, 46, 47
Protocols, 102–103, 111, 132
Proust, J., 110
Psychological insulin resistance, 19
Psychological self-monitoring, 110, 125
Psychology, ix, xvii, 84, 91, 92, 97, 104, 124
Public Reporting, 106, 111

## R

Randomized clinical trials, xv, xvii, 46, 56, 57, 60–62
Rational choice, 76, 85
Reach, G., ix, xi, xii, xvi, xvii
Regret, 84, 85, 87–91, 111, 112
Regulatory Focus Theory, 40–42, 89, 113
Reinforcement, 98, 105–109
Representativeness heuristic, 77
Risk, xii, xv, xvi, 1, 6, 9, 15, 18, 21–23, 32–34, 36, 39, 41, 54, 61–63, 75–76, 78–81, 83–86, 88, 89, 91, 92, 98, 99, 102, 106, 111, 113, 114, 122, 128, 131
Risk aversion, 78–79
Rogers, C., 90

## S

Sackett, D.L., 60
Scheen, A.J., 101
Schneewind, J.B., 126
Schön, D., 64–66, 68, 123, 130, 131
Schrödinger, E., 58–59, 84, 114
Searle, J., 74, 109, 129, 130
Sensitivity, 51–54, 77
Soft reasons, 32, 35
Specificity, 51–54, 77
Spinoza, B., 112–114
Statistical, 50, 54, 55, 57, 58, 75, 76, 80, 84, 123, 124
Straus, S.E., 60
Summerskill, W.S.P., 62, 82

# Index

**T**
Tappolet, C., 82, 132
Technical Rationality, 64, 65, 123
Telemedicine, 104–105
Test threshold, 52, 53
Therapeutic inertia, 6, 14, 15
Titration, 2, 15, 20, 21, 32, 35, 97, 98, 103
Tonelli, M.R., 62, 65, 132
Treatment threshold, 52, 53
True clinical inertia, 97–114, 132
Trust, xi, 35, 54, 113, 114, 124
Turner, B.J., 32, 33
Tversky, A., ix, 76, 78, 79, 88

**U**
Uncertainty, xii, 7, 20, 33, 34, 41, 50–56, 58,
    59, 63, 64, 66, 67, 75–78, 80, 91, 92,
    102–103, 106, 111, 114, 124–125, 131
Utility, 54, 55, 76, 78, 79, 85

**V**
Valvular heart disease, 22–23
Veazie, P.J., 41, 67, 89, 113

**W**
Wispé, L., 91

**Z**
Zajonc, R., 86